Catherine

FOR SHEILA
WITH LOVE
FROM ME
TO YOU

Julia Donaldson
xx

Also by the Author

A Fateful Rendezvous

Catherine

by
Julia Donal

Julia Donal • Liverpool

Copyright ©2012 Julia Donal

Book design and layout by MaryChris Bradley of The Book Team.

ISBN 978-1481986823 (trade paperback)

Contact the Author:
Email: julia6438@hotmail.com

To my husband Bill,
daughters Christine and Julianne,
and my son, Tony. Last, but by no means least,
to the memory of Catherine's father, Tony, Sr.

Catherine

There's a little girl who stayed when Alice came back home
And there's a small child in wonderland alone
She didn't mean to go away
She only left the house to play
And now she sits in silence
Sleeping in the stars at night in golden slumber breathing light
A lean gazelle that's taken fright, afraid, to come back home.

~ Poem written by Catherine's brother, Tony

Acknowledgements

THROUGHOUT THE five years that Catherine had been on programme; Bill and I wouldn't have been able to apply some of the special daily physical exercise's and many other tactile and other tasks that we had to do to help her, without the help and support of our family and many kind and caring people.

- My son Tony. My daughters, Christine and Julianne. Throughout the time, Bill and I were doing the Patterning programme with Catherine they may have felt I neglected them, which of course I never did and never would. What I want to say is that it could have been anyone of them on that terrible day in June 1972. I would have done exactly the same for them as I love them all equally, still do, and always will.

- To Bill's good friend Jacky who worked in the engineering department, of, The Metal Box Company in Speke, Liverpool. Every time we needed a new piece of equipment or special card so that we could make the flash cards, Jacky would approach his boss and explain what we were doing and why we were doing it. They always provided whatever we needed and never asked for anything in return; they just wished us well. Bill and I will never forget Jacky, who sadly passed away eight years ago and The Metal Box Company for their kindness and generosity and ongoing support when we need it.

- Not forgetting our friends, neighbours and family who supported us and helped us to raise enough money so we could begin the Doman Delacato Therapy.

- To Dot and George of Bridgewater, Somerset, who befriended three strangers, and who remained friends, even after Catherine had finished her programme. We wrote to each other until Dots death seven years ago.

- To my friend Michelle Daly, author of, *I Love Charlotte Brontë* and *With a Little Help from My Friends,* for her guidance, encouragement, help and advice.

- Last, but by no means least, my husband Bill, for no matter what obstacles we came up against regarding Catherine, and there have been many throughout the years, we have met them together. I thank him from the bottom of my heart for all the love, devotion and support he has given to me and Catherine. All I can say is that I have been truly blessed by having him beside me all these years.

Foreword

FROM NOWHERE the screams of my 11 year-old son Tony pierced the bright sunny afternoon. As I turned, he was running toward me with his arms out stretched and his eyes were bulging with terror. "Mum-Mum-come-quick, our Cathy's been run over" My heart was racing, pounding, as we both ran frantically back toward the road where a crowd of people were already gathered. I pushed my way through and couldn't believe what I saw before me. My little six-year-old daughter, my beautiful little girl was lying in the middle of the road. Blood was coming out of her nose and her ear. Her leg was bent halfway up her back and her eyes were tightly shut. I thought she was dead.

Part One

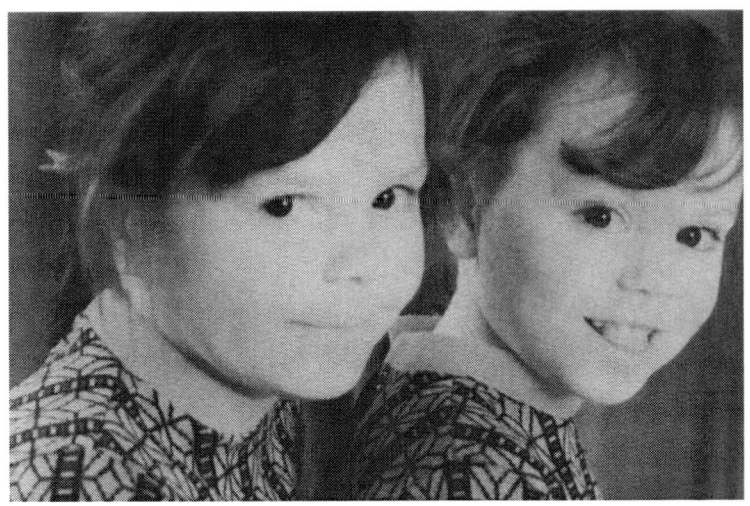

Catherine (on the right) with her sister Julianne, before the accident

~ 1 ~

A Day I Will Never Forget

MY HUSBAND was working as a caretaker at a school in the city and I had a part time job in Dunlop's from 5–9 in the evenings, not far from where we lived in Speke, on the outskirts of Liverpool. My job was a painter; which meant for four hours each evening I'd stand on a wooden palette and spray the bare golf balls with white paint as they came rolling down a Shute and onto a rotating machine which ensured that each golf ball was totally and evenly covered. However, before I could begin my job, I'd have to fill the Shute with the bare golf balls and hang my tin of white paint onto a large hook. Then, before I finished my shift, I'd have to clean my paint tin with Acetone. It was hard work.

The children were settled in school and so we went on day by day looking forward to the future as every family does; but it wasn't to be because fate was about to deal us a bitter and devastating blow.

Our eldest daughter Christine was a proper little lady and very particular about her appearance, going through the same ritual every morning. First, before she got dressed she'd inspect her clothes, just to make sure that I had ironed them properly. When she was satisfied, she'd get washed and dressed. Then before she left the house, she'd stand in front of the mirror over the fireplace and check her appearance as she brushed her fine strawberry blonde hair. Then she'd inspect her snow-white socks to ensure they were evenly matched around her ankles. Everything *had* to be neat and tidy. I looked at her with pride. She was growing into a lovely young woman. However, this particular day wasn't going to be like any other day–ever again.

Tony, our only son was a typical boy. Before he left the house each morning I'd have to grab him, just to make sure that soap and water had connected with his neck. He was a happy, affectionate and mischievous child and so full of fun. He loved football and was captain of his team. However, that day my son was about to witness something, the memory of which, would be etched in his mind for the rest of his life

It was good that Christine and Tony could see to themselves because I had two younger daughters to attend to, Julianne, at eight years old, was a bonny little girl and very outgoing, with many friends both in and out of school. She was self-conscious about her smile having lost a few of her baby teeth. Sometimes the boys would call for her to play football—she played mid-field and a good one at that.

My youngest, Catherine had just had her sixth birthday on June 17th. She, like her sister Julianne, loved playing outdoors. Sometimes in the evenings, they'd have a concert and they would take turns to sing. If one sang for longer than the other did, an argument would start and I'd have to break it up. Julianne would go outside to sulk and Catherine would sit inside and sulk but after a couple of minutes she'd run outside looking for her sister, the argument forgotten.

My children my beautiful children—were growing up fast. Their father and I were so proud of them.

It was the 28th June 1972. This was the day that my son Tony, and many others were about to be confirmed by the Archbishop of Liverpool. There was an air of excitement in the school and lots of pomp and ceremony in the church.

I'd bought Tony a new shirt and trousers. He was such a handsome boy and I wanted him to look his best.

However, that day, from the moment I climbed out of bed, a dark cloud hung over me. I tried to ignore it but I couldn't. That afternoon, I was on the open-green helping my sister-in-law look after my sister's three under-five tots whilst she was in hospital.

Then from nowhere, the screams of my 11year-old son Tony, pierced the bright sunny afternoon. As I turned, he was running toward me with his arms outstretched and his eyes bulging with terror.

"Mum! Mum! Come quick, our Cathy's been run over"

My heart was racing, pounding, as Tony and I ran frantically back toward the road where I could see a crowd of people already gathered. I pushed my way through and couldn't believe what I saw. My six-year-old little girl, my beautiful little Catherine was lying in the middle of the road with blood coming out of her nose and ear. With her leg bent halfway up her back and her eyes tightly shut, I thought she was dead!

That terrible feeling of foreboding that I had had all that day had come to fruition. Nothing would ever be the same again. We were about to enter a dark and unavoidable void. My nightmare had begun.

Our Living Nightmare Begins

I BENT down to where Catherine lay, and was about to take her in my arms when I was restrained by some of the parents at the scene. A woman I didn't recognise looked at me pitifully and said "Don't touch her love, you could make her worse"

"Let go of me," I screamed. I tried to fight them off but my arms were being held so firmly that I couldn't move them. I dropped my head in despair and sobbed as I looked at the body of my baby lying helpless and injured on the road. Then a woman shouted from the crowd, "Don't worry love the ambulance is on its way." As the grip loosened on my arms, I managed to pull away. Then a man I knew stood in front of me with his arms outstretched as he tried to stop me from picking her up. I pulled and struggled to free myself from his grasp. I felt I had the strength of ten men; I desperately wanted to hold my child.

The sound of the siren brought me to my senses as the ambulance arrived and my caring captors released me.

Two paramedics jumped from the ambulance, opened the back doors and brought out a stretcher. I watched them crouch down on the tarmac and gently place the tiny lifeless body of my little girl upon it. Then they placed her on the narrow bed inside their vehicle. I followed anxiously behind as my neighbour shouted to me "Don't worry about the kids, love, I'll keep an eye on them. Someone has sent for Catherine's father and he's on his way." With my eyes glued firmly on my baby, I couldn't answer her. The ambulance doors slammed shut and one of the ambulance men remained in the back with us. I was so devastated. Throughout our stressful journey, he kept reassuring me that a team of the best doctors were waiting for her at the hospital and would do their very best for Catherine.

The emergency siren blasted all the way to the children's hospital in Myrtle Street, shooting through red traffic lights in a desperate bid to save my daughter's life. I knelt down beside her on the floor of the ambulance and held her tiny lifeless hand.

AT LUNCHTIME that day, I walked up to school as usual to bring Catherine home for lunch. I'd just been to the shop to buy her a small custard tart, which was her favourite. She was going to have it after she'd eaten her lunch. As I walked home, I held the small paper bag containing her treat. Then suddenly I felt so emotional my eyes filled with tears. I quickened my step. I needed to get back home. I kept muttering to myself. "Oh dear God, what's wrong with me?"

Catherine and I sat at the little kitchen table together. She told me what she had been doing in school that morning. She was a bright little girl, could read and write and had accumulated a few gold stars in the short time since she started school. As she chatted, I couldn't take my eyes off her. I couldn't understand why I felt the way I did.

After Catherine had eaten her cheese sandwiches she said, "I don't feel like my custard tart right now mum, I'll leave it till I come home"

"That's ok," I said and put the custard tart in the fridge. Then she ran upstairs to wash her hands and face. When she came down, she said, "I think I'll go back to school now mum, my friends will be waiting for me." She smiled at me and I put my arms around her and held her close. That terrible feeling had come over me again.

We walked back to school together. When we got to the playground, she ran toward her friends who were waiting for her. She looked back and waved to me and shouted "Bye Mum, see you after." I waved back to her and walked slowly away. Little did I know that that would be the last time she would ever be able to speak to me I had promised that she could come home from school with her friends at half past three. She wanted to bring school friends home just like her older sister Julianne did.

My son Tony would be home earlier from school that day to prepare for his Confirmation in the evening. I told him to meet Catherine on the corner at half past three and that she'd have her friends with her. I was comfortable with this arrangement because there was a lollipop man in attendance to cross them over the road.

Those two hours passed quickly as Betty and I played with my sister's children, but even those little children couldn't distract me from that terrible feeling which had gnawed at my brain all day. Then my son's screams pierced the air.

WHEN WE arrived at the hospital, a medical team had been standing by to meet us. The ambulance men flung open the doors and lifted my unconscious child out on the stretcher. Gentle hands transferred her to a trolley and they quickly rushed her into the examination room. They wouldn't let me go with her. No matter how much I pleaded with them, they wouldn't allow me to follow. A nurse took hold of my arm and ushered me gently into a small waiting room, which was adjacent to the examination room. She looked on helplessly as I paced the waiting room floor. When I did sit down my hands were gripping my hair as I rocked my head back and forth out of my mind with worry.

Then I heard my husband's voice. He was asking where Catherine and I were. The nurse brought him in to me and we just looked at one another too grief stricken to speak. Then he walked toward me and we held each other tight, united in the fear and uncertainty of whether our beautiful daughter was going to live or die.

Soon a doctor came into the room and gave us his diagnosis. He said that Catherine had suffered multiple and appalling injuries. Her condition was very serious and they would have to operate straight away. He asked us to sign a consent form, which we did without any hesitation. We would do anything to save our little girl.

I don't know how long Catherine's father and I sat silently together in the tiny antiseptic waiting room, each nursing our own fears. We were told when other members of the family had arrived but we didn't see them because they were taken to another room.

Then our silence was broken when a nurse came in and asked Tony and I to follow her. She took us upstairs and showed us into another waiting room. It was the waiting room for ward 5, where Catherine would come from the operating theatre.

So, we waited and waited. The longer the wait the more anxious we became. Then at last—it was about eight o'clock in the evening—when the doctor came into the room. We could tell by the look on his face that it wasn't good news. We sprang out of our seats to greet him, desperate to hear what he was going to say.

Then he asked us to sit down and as we did, we never took our eyes off him. "I'm afraid your daughter's condition is very serious," he said sympathetically. "She has suffered severe head injuries resulting in irreparable damage to her brain. The femur in her right leg is broken and all we can do now is to make her as comfortable as possible. She may not survive the night but if she does, the next 24 hours will be crucial. I suggest that you inform the rest of your family. I'm sure they would like to see her."

I stared at him. I couldn't believe what he was saying. He said that our beautiful, bright, mischievous little girl was probably going to die. But he didn't know her; he must be mistaken. Doctors always say these terrible things. They always paint things darker than they really are. "No! No! No!" I screamed. "You're wrong. I don't believe you." I began clawing at the walls trying to escape the words I no longer wanted to hear; escape from the horrifying reality of the situation. Tony put his arms around me and tears were running down his face. He cupped my face in his hands, looked at me and said, "We've just got to wait and see. They don't know her like we do, do they love?"

Just then, a staff nurse came into the room. She held a small glass of water in her hand and a white tablet in the other. She offered them to me and said, "Please, please take this. It will help you. You'll be going to see Catherine soon and I'm sure she wouldn't like to see her mum so upset."

The doctor looked at us both and said, "I'll be back in just a moment."

Tony turned his tear-stained face to me and said, "Please love, take it, it will make you feel better."

I protested, "I don't want any drugs. I don't want to be put to sleep. I just want my little girl."

"I promise it's not to make you sleep. It's just to steady your nerves," the nurse said kindly.

I looked at my husband and he nodded his head; so I took the tablet and gladly drank the water; my throat was so dry.

When the doctor returned, he had a ward sister with him. "This is Sister Western," he said. "She will take you to see Catherine. She's ready for you now. She's nice and comfortable and all tucked up in bed. You will see a small machine at the side of her bed, which is just to help her to breathe. Her head is bandaged and very swollen and that's because of her injuries, but I promise you that day by day her head will get back to its normal size so don't be too alarmed. We will be monitoring her condition constantly and will do so for as long as it takes. I'm going to leave you now in the capable hands of Sister Western. She will look after you both. If there is anything that you want to know or are anxious about please ask. I will have to go now, I'm wanted downstairs. I will see you again sometime tomorrow." He smiled at us both said good-bye and left.

~ 3 ~

Touch and Go

"CATHERINE'S WARD'S just here," Sister Western said. She pushed open the dark red swing doors and walked silently and swiftly past the tiny beds that stood on both sides the ward, her starched uniform swishing quietly in her wake. The third bed on the right had curtains drawn around it. Sister Western drew back the curtains, looked at us both and smiled saying, "Here she is. Here's Catherine." A dim light from the bedside lamp shone gently upon the small and lifeless body of our little girl swaddled in bandages. At the side of the bed was a machine that made rhythmical puffing sounds as the pump went up and down.

"Don't be alarmed the machine is helping her to breath." Sister Western gently cautioned, "It's allowing Catherine to rest and she needs plenty of rest for what she's been through. I am going to leave you both for a little while. I will be in the office if you need me." She put her hand on my arm and said, "I'm sure you both could do with a cup of tea, I'll organise it." She half smiled and gave us a pitiful look before quickly walking away.

Catherine's father and I stood on either side of her bed in complete silence. The tiny figure on the bed looked nothing like Catherine. Her bandaged head seemed to have to have swollen to twice its natural size. Her forehead and eyelids were black and blue; her very swollen leg was in an iron cast because her femur had been broken. I reached down and clutched her tiny hand in mine. Tony was leaning on the bed with his head bowed silently sobbing. An air of utter despair came over us. Our baby daughter was going to die there was nothing we could do to help her.

The cubicle curtain swished open as Sister Western came in and placed a small tray on the bedside table with two mugs of hot tea. She sat with us for a while and chatted, doing her best to reassure us that everything that could be done was being done. She said they would be monitoring her condition constantly and would keep her as comfortable as possible. A staff nurse breezed in and out of the curtains every fifteen minutes or so monitoring Catherine's temperature. After an hour or so sister Western said that maybe it would be a good idea if we went home and told Catherine's brother and sisters how ill their little sister was.

After reassuring us, that Catherine would be in safe hands, we left, but our hearts were heavy with despair. We got a taxi outside the hospital and made our way home. We were eager to see our children; but we were not looking forward to what we had to tell them.

Christine, Tony junior and Julianne were alright; my neighbour and good friend Hilda had been keeping watch over them, but understandably, they were anxious to hear news of their little sister. Between us, their father and I tried to explain to them how ill Catherine was. We couldn't tell them the awful truth of how serious her injuries were and with sadness in all our hearts we sent them off to bed.

I went into the kitchen to make a cup of tea. As I opened the fridge to get the milk, the custard tart was still there. I took it out and threw it against the kitchen wall. The pain was so unbearable I felt as if my heart was bleeding. My husband and I stayed up all night. We couldn't go to bed; sleep was impossible.

In the meantime, my neighbour, whose son was having his confirmation at the same time as my son told me her husband had taken my son Tony with them to the church and had him confirmed as well. I was so grateful for that. I didn't want my son to miss out on his Confirmation.

Throughout the night, we prayed and drank tea; eagerly waiting for morning to come so that when the children had gone to school, we could leave for the hospital. Every hour on the hour Catherine's father went to the phone box on the corner of the road and rang Sister Western. There was no change.

At last, morning came and after seeing that all was well with the children or as well as could expected under the circumstances, we prepared to leave for the hospital. The children were going to Masie's, their father's cousin, straight from school for their tea. Masie had moved into our area a couple of years previously. Before we left for the hospital, we rang Sister Western. She said Catherine's condition had worsened slightly and she was critical.

When we arrived at the hospital, the doctor was waiting for us in Sister Western's office. He told us that he had taken Catherine off the breathing machine because she had begun to breathe for herself. Unfortunately that was all she could do. Her condition had deteriorated and could turn fatal at anytime. She had also slipped into a coma.

He said Catherine could stay that way for weeks, months or even years. This news was far too much for us to bear; it was living nightmare. The thoughts of losing our little girl left us both with a feeling of hopelessness.

I wanted to run out onto the street and scream "Help us please somebody help us, our little girl is dying!"

We put our arms around each other and cried desperately. Then a cloud of despair covered me and I slid through his arms to the floor. If Catherine was going to die then I was going with her. She was too young and too little to die alone. The suffering was unbearable. Oh God what would life be like without her? All of our four children were so very precious to us.

~ 4 ~

Our Bedside Vigil

AFTER OUR tears subsided, although there were many more to come, we had to decide what we were going to do. There was no way we would leave Catherine on her own in a coma; one of us would have to be there to talk to her and let her know that we were right beside her. However, we had three other children at home who needed us and they were suffering as well. We were a unit of six but one was missing so we were incomplete. We decided that I would stay with Catherine in the daytime and her father would stay with her throughout the night. That way one of us would be there if the worst came to the worst. The hospital gave us a parent's room, which consisted of basic essentials, two single beds and facilities to make a cup of tea. It was 1972.

With a heavy heart, I left Catherine's father sitting beside her bed and made my way to the bus stop around the corner from the hospital. There were many young students from Liverpool University waiting for the bus; I presumed all were making their way back to their respective bed-sits. I leaned against the brick wall, watched, and listened. Some were laughing, some were talking and some were making plans for the evening. Others were complaining about the amount of homework they had to do. As I listened, sadness filled my heart. My spirit was broken. According to the doctors, Catherine would never enjoy independence like these students. I wanted to tell these young happy fun-loving teenagers that my child was dying. I wanted to tell them how alone and desperate I felt, but they wouldn't understand. How could they? They had the world at their feet and were aiming to leave their mark and rightly so. It was now a world that had been denied to our precious daughter; but it wasn't their fault that Catherine was dying.

Then shouts of "Here comes the bus!" interrupted my troubled thoughts and brought me back to my senses and I climbed aboard. I don't remember the journey back home. My mind was totally occupied with what, and how I was going to tell Christine, young Tony, and Julianne about their sister. How would they cope without her? *Please God help me. What am I going to tell them?* I arrived home before the children. I took off my coat and shoes and left them in a crumpled heap at the bottom of the stairs; then I ran upstairs, went into my bedroom, got down on my knees, and prayed.

"Please God help our little girl, wrap your loving arms around her and hold her close to your heart, please don't let her die—we need her so much. The doctor at the hospital said that even if she comes out of the coma she will be badly brain damaged and that she will always need looking after and she will never be able to do anything for herself. Please God don't let her die. I don't care what's wrong with her, we will always look after her. Please God don't punish her for my sins—take me instead" My prayers were interrupted by a knock on the front door. I ran down stairs and opened it.

My daughter Julianne and her friend where standing in the path. She looked up at me and said "Hiya mum how's our Cathy? Is she better? When can we see her? The whole of our school and all the other schools in Speke have been saying prayers for her"

My voice faltered but I tried to put on a brave face and said "Wait till Christine and Tony come home and I'll tell you all together" As soon as the others came home their first question was of course, "How's our Cathy mum?"

Before I could answer, I took a deep breath, tried to keep the quiver out of my voice, and told them the best way I could.

I said that her condition was serious and that we would all have to pray very hard. I explained to them what their father and I had decided; that I would stay with Catherine during the day, but also stressed to them that I would be here for them when they came home from school. Their father would be with Catherine at night so that she wouldn't be left alone. Knowing that one of us would be with their little sister at all times, seemed to help them. Then they wanted to know when they could see her. I promised that as soon as her condition improves we would take them to the hospital for a visit. I didn't want them to see the tiny grotesque figure that was their little sister, Catherine lying lifeless on a hospital bed. Yet, if she wasn't going to make it we had no option but to let them visit. We would have to take them into the hospital to see her.

No phone call during the night. We didn't have a phone of our own and rang the ward from a public call box on the corner of the road. However, if Catherine's condition worsened the hospital would get in touch with our local police and they would come and let me know, but I couldn't settle. Throughout the night, while my children slept I paced the living room floor, drank endless cups of coffee and smoked the last two cigarettes I had left.

As I looked out of the window into the darkness of the night my eyes were drawn to the road where just a short time ago my little girl had lain. Tears began to fall silently. Oh, God I whispered, "Why did this awful thing happen to us?"

As dawn broke, the early morning sun filled the living room with light. I went into the kitchen and made myself a cup of tea. The children would be up soon wanting their breakfast. I was eager to get to the hospital, eager to see what was happening. After breakfast we said our goodbyes and the children went off to school with the understanding I would be there waiting when they came home.

I left hurriedly. I wanted to catch the Crossville bus, which stopped right outside the little Polish Catholic Church of St Philip Neri in Catherine Street.

~ 5 ~

Torn Between my Children

I GOT off the bus at the stop before the hospital and went into the Catholic Church of Saint Philip Neri, which was visible from the hospital. I dipped my fingers into the font and blessed myself with holy water. To the right of the font and just inside a small alcove there stood a statue of Saint Jude. My aunt had told me he was the patron saint of hopeless causes. I knelt on the tiny wooden support, clasped my hands together and looked pleadingly into the face of the image of Saint Jude. With an aching heart, I begged Saint Jude to intercede for me to Almighty God. I wanted him to ask God to spare Catherine, to let her live. "We don't care what's wrong with her," I whispered. "We will always look after her. Just please—please—don't let her die!"

After my sorrowful prayers, I took the short walk to the hospital, hoping against all hope that a miracle would have happened. I pictured the scene in my mind. It would be like this: I would walk into the ward and my husband, Tony would be standing there with his arms outstretched to me, a big smile on his face and he'd say. "Catherine's awake! She's awake—and asking for you." Then Catherine would look at me and say, "Hiya mum, when can I come home." Of course, that was all in my imagination, because when I walked into the ward Catherine was lying in the same position, on her back with her eyes tightly closed.

Usually when I arrived at the hospital Catherine's father would leave. He'd be exhausted after sitting at Catherine's bedside all night. Day after day, it was the same routine. I felt total and utter despair; but my daughter was still alive and holding her own so there was still hope.

One day when I walked into the ward, Sister Western was standing beside Catherine's bed. She greeted me with a smile and said, "Her breathing is steady, she's had a bed bath and I've made her nice and comfortable.

"Sit and talk to her; talk about anything she could relate to, talk about her brother and sisters, your neighbours, people she knows."

About four weeks after the accident the doctor who was looking after Catherine called us into his office. He said as far her condition was concerned she could stay like that for some time. Sadly, he just couldn't say if or when she would ever wake up, but for us to rest assured, she was in safe hands and would be cared for no matter how long as it took.

He continued to say that it would be better for our sakes and the welfare of our other children if we could try to get some sort of normality back into our lives if that was at all possible.

We knew what he'd said made sense yet we were so torn. It was heartbreaking; we didn't want to leave her but we had our other children to think about and they needed us too. So we arranged for me to visit during the afternoon and Catherine's father could call in from work. The school where he worked was a fifteen-minute walk from the hospital. If there were, any serious developments during our absence the hospital would get in touch with us right away.

Weeks turned into months and I went to the hospital every afternoon, always making sure I was home for the children when they returned from school.

In the meantime the constant stress of travelling to the hospital every day to see Catherine, and then having to leave her so I could catch the bus and be home for the children coming in from school, was exhausting. Then, lying in bed at night dreading a knock on the door from the police to tell us Catherine's condition had worsened.

I couldn't return to work and my husband lost his job because he'd taken so much time off, so our finances were stretched, to say the least. Things went from bad to worse, after seeking legal advice, it was determined Catherine had sustained her terrible injuries through an accident and the lorry-driver's firm accepted no responsibility. My daughter never even got so much as a card or a bar of chocolate from them.

~ 6 ~

Elation

CATHERINE HAD lain in a coma for six long agonising months. During that time, her hair had grown back but it was darker and thicker than it used to be. Her bruising had cleared, there were no bandages and the iron was off her leg. She looked just like a little girl who had fallen asleep, until the morning of the 19 Dec 72, when her father and I walked into the hospital together.

Sister Western and the parish priest from Saint Philip Neri where standing around Catherine's bed. We walked quickly toward them.

Sister Western looked at us with a beaming smile and said, "Look, she's coming out of the coma. I've sent for the doctor and he's on his way."

Her father and I looked at one another in disbelief and our faces glowed with happiness. We were elated and so full of joy I felt as if I was going burst. I looked at my husband and said, "Wait till we tell the kid's they'll be made up. This is going to be our best Christmas ever."

The doctor walked briskly into the ward eager to see what was happening to his little patient. He stood at the foot of her bed and looked at her; then he smiled and said, "Hello Catherine, how are you? It's lovely to see you." She just stared blankly at him.

He walked around the bed and shone a pencil slim light into her eyes and placed his stethoscope on her chest. After he'd finished his brief examination he looked at both of us and said, "She's in a comatose condition at the moment. The best thing to do is to talk to her and keep talking to her, just as you've been doing all this time. I'm going to get in touch with a specialist from Alder Hey Children's Hospital to ask for an assessment of her condition and if anything can be done for her…I'm afraid that it will be sometime after Christmas before we can have her assessed"

We nodded our approval. We didn't mind waiting till after Christmas. We'd waited six long agonizing months for this day. We were so excited our little girl was coming around. If we could get back to where we were before this tragedy happened, we'd be complete again. We couldn't wait to tell her brother and sisters.

We sat either side of Catherine's bed and held her hand. She looked at us with a vacant stare; she was just like a new baby. I stood up and slowly walked around to the other side of the bed to where her father was sitting and put my hand on his shoulder. She followed me with her eyes but there were no signs of recognition. At that moment, we didn't care what she could do or couldn't do because she'd been so ill. She'd been in a coma all that time so for the moment what could we expect?

Then I felt as if something strange had happened. It was as if a quiet sense of freedom and relief had come over us both. I felt as if the past six months had slipped away and a very large and heavy millstone had been lifted from our shoulders.

When we got home later that day, we told our children the good news. Of course the first thing that they wanted to know was when could they see her and when was she coming home? We had taken them into the hospital to see her but not till the bruising and swelling had gone down. We explained what the doctor had said. That before she could come home a special doctor was coming to see her but it wouldn't be till after Christmas. Then we hoped he would tell us when she could come home, and how we could help her.

But we can all be with her on Christmas day and spend the day together; Something a couple of months ago we thought would be impossible.

There were other families spending Christmas day at the hospital because some of the children were very ill. Several of the tiny patients had been born with heart defects.

On Christmas day, Christine, Tony Junior, Julianne, her father and I all sat around Catherine's bed. As each one of us spoke to her, she just looked at us; and there were no signs of recognition or communication. She just lay there propped up with pillows.

When the nurse came to change her there were no sounds of protest and her arms and legs flopped just like a rag doll. Still, for all she had been through she was a picture of beauty. Her dark thick hair curled around her face. Her eyes though dull were tinted green and her skin was smooth and pink. She was indeed, although awake, a sleeping beauty.

The New Year began with no great improvement in her condition. She couldn't take food by mouth so she had to be fed by a tube.

The nurse would gently push a thin tube though Catherine's nostril and into her stomach. Then feed her an amount of special liquid through the tube by a large hypodermic like syringe. I told Sister Western I didn't like Catherine having that tube pushed though her nose. She explained that the tube feeding Catherine was called an oesophageal tube and the reason she was being fed that way was because she wasn't able to swallow and it was the only way they could feed her. She also said that before Catherine could come home, I would have to learn the procedure. I panicked. I told her that I couldn't possibly do that.

She replied, "Of course you can because I'm going to teach you. You won't be placing the tube yourself of course the district nurse will do that. I am going to show you how to feed Catherine once the nurse had placed the tube.

It didn't take me long to learn how to feed Catherine from the tube; under the watchful eye of Sister Western or the staff nurse. I was very apprehensive about doing it, but also very relieved that the district nurse would be calling at least four times a week to change and check the tube. About a week later, I told Sister Western that I felt confident and I was ready to feed Catherine myself from the tube. It was then she arranged for the specialist to come and assess her. I was desperate to have her back home to be with her family.

The day for Catherine's assessment was the 5th February 1973. Her father and I sat nervously beside her bed waiting for the specialist to arrive. Then we saw him. Well, we presumed it was him, because he walked onto the ward with an air of importance. He wore a smart dark suit and carried a black briefcase. He went into sister's office at the entrance to the ward. We could see him and sister talking together then she handed him a file, which he opened and read briefly. They both came out of the office and walked toward us. Sister Western introduced him as a child specialist from Alder Hey Children's Hospital Liverpool.

He looked at us both and nodded his head in acknowledgment. Then he pursed his lips together and stood for a little while at the bottom of Catherine's bed just looking at her and then at last, he proceeded with his assessment.

He looked deeply into her eyes with his special torch and when he pinched her hands and feet, she moved slightly. He examined her chest and looked in her ears.

As he straightened himself up he sighed deeply and shook his head from side to side; then he looked at her father and I and said coldly.

"The best advice that I can give you both is, go home and take care of the three children you have. The kindest thing that you can do for this child, is to have her placed in some kind of care home and let someone else take care of her.

"She will never be able to do anything for herself and will always have to depend on someone. She will never walk, talk or be able to feed herself.

"All in all she will be totally dependent on others for the rest of her life. She will always be in nappies and as far as her quality of life is concerned, it will be non-existent."

Her father and I were shocked and angry at the way he had spoken. It wasn't about the result of the assessment, it was about his cold and condescending attitude and the way he'd spoken about Catherine. Her father stared at the doctor and I could see his fists clenched. I put my hand on his arm to restrain him and said quietly "We're not going to take any notice of him. Just wait till we get her back home, we'll get her better, just wait and see." Then the specialist picked up his briefcase from the chair, nodded to us and walked away with Sister Western following in swift pursuit.

After the child specialist had gone, Sister Western came to see us. She didn't make any comment on what the doctor had said. She just said that she was going to arrange for Catherine's long awaited return home.

We arrived early at the hospital on the 6 Feb 1973 where an ambulance was waiting for us to bring Catherine home. The ambulance men propped her up in a sitting position on a stretcher. Sister Western came to the entrance of the hospital to see us off and handed me an appointment card. We were to take Catherine back to see the doctor in three month's time to see what, if any, progress she had made. Sister Western was a great comfort to me during the long months Catherine had been in hospital. Sometimes when she was on duty, when I came to visit Catherine, I would find her sitting at the side of Catherine's bed talking to her; then when I'd walk in and I would sit on the bed and join in the conversation; she was so supportive to me and my husband during those long and lonely months and never stopped encouraging us to have hope. I will never forget Sister Western.

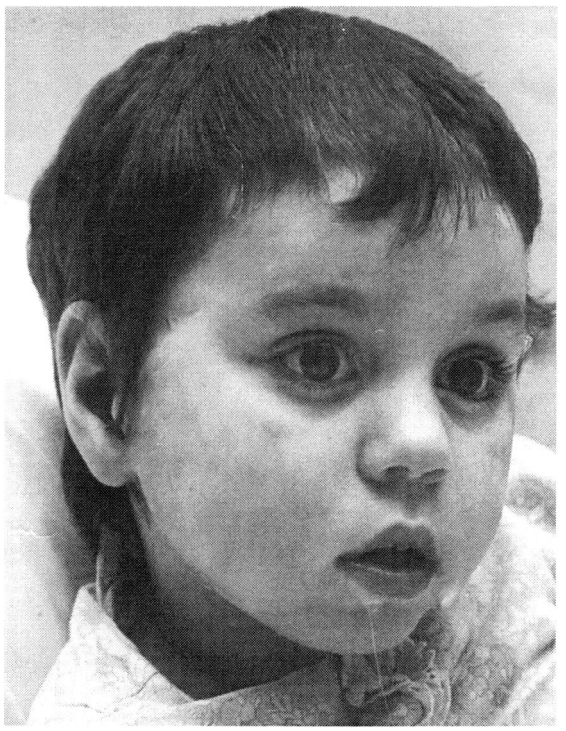

Catherine, finally awake after being in a coma for six months

Our Campaign Begins

MY DAUGHTER had been in hospital from 28th June 1972 until 6th Feb 1973. A district nurse was to call every day to check her feeding tube and report on any progress that Catherine might make.

So we arrived back home. Her father carried her into the front room and I propped her up with a couple of pillows' on the settee.

She was all ready and waiting for her brother and sisters to come home from school. They duly arrived and were elated to see their little sister again. It didn't matter to them that she couldn't put her arms about them; they put their arms tightly around her. They just saw her as we saw her, she was our Cathy and she was back in the fold again.

Her father and I knew deep down that this was going to be an uphill struggle. We were ready to take the challenge. We were going to take it day by day.

As Catherine lay in a deep coma and in between hospital visits, her father and I, a group of friends and some of our neighbours, themselves parents, decided to campaign for a Zebra crossing to be placed in Western Avenue, where Catherine had been knocked down. We arranged a meeting at our house. We agreed, that to bring attention to our cause we would block off Western Avenue and join hands at the exact spot where Catherine had been knocked down.

The day after our meeting, Catherine's father and I and other parents stood in the middle of the road, joined hands and blocked off the intended spot. The build-up of traffic was awful. Some motorists were shouting to us to get out of the way, but we held on to each other tightly and didn't budge. In no time at all, the police came. The police officer in charge said, what we were doing was an unlawful, dangerous act and if we didn't disperse Catherine's father would be arrested. This caused some anger, so much so, that some of the people who were watching us joined us in the protest. We all gathered around my husband and made it perfectly clear to the police that if they were going to arrest him they would have to arrest us all.

There was no shouting or anything like that. A peaceful protest was what we needed and we wanted to keep it that way, but it did cause havoc and it did bring attention to our cause. The police were adamant and said we would have to end our protest because as far as they (the police) were concerned we had made our stand. Eventually we made an agreement with the police to end our protest for the time being at least. The police officer in charge accompanied my husband and I back to our house.

We told him why were campaigning and how seriously ill Catherine was. After listening patiently and sympathetically to what we said. He told us our protest was wrong, especially when there is a build up of traffic, making the situation quite dangerous. He said that the proper way to go about getting things done was to write to the council and tell them about Catherine's accident; and how it had affected all the other parents whose children use the same road to get to and from school.

What he said made sense, so a couple of days later we had a meeting and I wrote a letter to the council about our campaign and why. We said that we would like a meeting as soon as possible to see what could be done about the busy junction in Western Avenue. Although there was a crossing attendant, he was an elderly man and the situation needed looking at as soon as possible. About four weeks later, we received a letter from the council   accompanied with a time and date informing us that an official from the council was coming to see us with a representative from the police. We were prepared and ready to hear what they had to say.

The man from the council was polite but very forthright. He said that while he totally understood how Catherine's father and I and the other parents felt, he didn't really think it was necessary to put a Zebra Crossing in Western Avenue and furthermore, if they did place a Zebra Crossing in Western Avenue other parts of Speke will start campaigning for one. It was blatantly obvious that he was thinking about the cost. We told him that our children were priceless and as far as the cost of a Zebra Crossing was concerned, there was no comparison. We also told him that we would keep up our protest until something was resolved.

The police representative wasn't very happy with our reaction. After a couple of hours of intense arguments of the pros and cons, I must say that there were more 'for' than 'against.'

The man from the council said that it wasn't up to him to say if a meeting could be arranged with the council to discuss the matter further; but he would most certainly do his best to put our case forward at the next council meeting. He added that we would have to be patient because the next council meeting would be in about six week's time and he promised that we would receive letter regarding the outcome.

We waited till the six weeks had passed and there was no word regarding the outcome of the council meeting. My husband and I and our supporters were about to start another protest by blocking off the road again when a letter from the council arrived.

Firstly, the letter said that they were very sorry to hear about Catherine's accident and hoped that she would make a full recovery. It also said that the council had taken notes about our protest regarding the Zebra Crossing. They were going to arrange a meeting with the highways committee where our appeal for a Zebra Crossing could be discussed in depth; and this meeting would take place in about four weeks time.

In the meantime, they (the council) would be sending a surveyor to look at the road were the accident had happened and would wait on his findings. All this was going to take time, we were to be patient, and they guaranteed that they would write to us when they had gathered all the needed information that.

After more than three years of corresponding back and forth with the council, we received the letter regarding the Zebra Crossing, it said. After much deliberation, they, Liverpool City Council decided there were grounds to place a Zebra Crossing at the junction in Western Avenue, Blackrod Avenue, and Stapleton Avenue as there were five schools using that particular junction every day. In addition, as it was a fast growing population, it would be advisable to place a Zebra Crossing at the suggested sight.

To say we were delighted would be an understatement. It didn't make any difference to Catherine's injuries and it wouldn't make her any better, but at least it may prevent another terrible tragedy

About a year later, work began on the crossing. It pleases me to see parents taking their children on the Zebra Crossing as they go back and forth to school each day. Even though its forty years since Catherine's accident; I do my best to avoid driving up Western Avenue because I still see the place where my little girl had lain. The Zebra Crossing will always be a reminder of what had happened on that terrible day 28 June 1972. Not that my family or I could ever forget because it will be with us until the day we die.

~ 8 ~

A Family Once Again

IT WAS good to have Catherine home again, no more travelling backward and forward to the hospital every day. We tried our best to be as we were before; but her father and I knew that things would never be the same again.

The first thing that concerned me was her sleeping arrangements. When she was in hospital, she slept in a bed with adjustable sides that pulled up or down so there was no fear of her falling out. A friend of mine had a large wooden cot that her youngest child had grown too big for it so she gave it to me; it was just what I needed because it had an adjustable side. We put the cot into the bedroom that she shared with her two sisters, Christine and Julianne. My son Tony had his own room.

I was a bit nervous when we first brought her home because she had the feeding tube taped to her cheek. She was also in nappies and her limbs were still slightly stiff and not very supple. However, she would have physiotherapy at the hospital, once a week. The physiotherapist was going to show her father and I what we were to do and how we were to do it.

The first morning was the scariest. After the children had gone to school and her father had left for work I was on my own. The first task would be to bathe her. I filled the bath half-full of warm water and added a foaming bath cube. Then I laid out a change of clothes for her on my bed. I went into the bedroom pushed down the side of the cot and lifted her out. Even though she was a petite little girl, she was six years and eight months old. I carried her into the bathroom. As I placed her gently into the warm water, she closed her eyes. As I splashed the warm water slowly over her tired, little body I began to sing one of the songs that she used to sing.

"Sunday morning up with the lark think I'll take a walk in the park, hey, hey it's a beautiful day."

There was also Findus fish advert on the television which she liked because she loved the tune it was called "Gone fishing gone away" accompanied by a short film of a fishing trawler. One of my neighbours wrote to Findus.

She explained how ill Catherine was and she was in a coma and we were looking for anything that we could do that might bring her round. Findus were very kind and sent us a recording of the song and the name of the singer, which was Jane Relf.

As I sang to her, she gave me a lovely smile, which made me wonder had she remembered the song; on the other hand, it could be that she loved the soothing effects of the water. After a short while, I lifted her out of the bath, placed her on my knee, and wrapped a big bath towel around her.

I carried her into my bedroom. I had to get her dressed because the district nurse would be calling soon. I laid her down on the bed, powdered her all over, and applied cream onto her bottom. Then I cut a piece of padding from a large reel that the district nurse had given me to use as nappies. I dressed her in one of her favourite things a pink hand-knitted little suit; it was February and it would keep her nice and warm. I brushed her thick dark hair, which had begun to curl around her face. Her beautiful eyes were speckled grey and green and her dark lashes were long and curled; she looked a little picture. As I lifted her up into my arms and held her close to me, hot tears began to run down my cheeks. I've never been a religious person but I began to cry bitterly and called out loudly. "Please God help me; show me what to do." I had no one else to turn to.

After I had composed myself, I carried Catherine down stairs, took her into the front room and placed her on the settee. Then I propped her into a sitting position with some pillows so that she could look out of the window and watch the large willow tree; which stood in my next-door neighbour's front garden, as it swayed back and forth from the force of the bitter winter wind.

Having left her securely propped up on the settee I ran up stairs to wash my face and comb my hair before the district nurse came. As I brushed my hair, I stopped and stared at the face that looked back at me and thought how old I looked. The stresses of the last few months were beginning to take their toll. I was thirty-four years old but I looked much older. As I turned away from the mirror, a thought occurred to me of how I was to cope with Catherine's daily needs. Do exactly what you did each time you brought a new baby home start from the very beginning! I felt as if a light had gone on in my head. Thank you God, for answering my prayers!

9

Standing My Ground

FOR THE first few weeks, that Catherine had been out of hospital the district nurse called every day and I was very grateful because I was still a little nervous about feeding her through the tube. I knew that it was a necessity but I thought it was unnatural.

After greeting each other every morning she'd always ask the same questions like, "Did Catherine sleep well? Had I slept well," well the answer to that would be, "no I hadn't; I very rarely did because I'm always on the alert just in case Catherine chokes." As we talked, I told her that slowly but surely, in fact I knew that Catherine had begun to improve because her eyes were much brighter and she was taking more notice of her surroundings and watching all that was going on. She replied that she was very pleased to hear it; but I really don't think she believed me.

Then after our little chitchat, she would change Catherine's tube and write in her notebook. I hated that tube so much. I know that Catherine never liked it either because she used to balk each time the nurse inserted a new one.

One morning, after thinking long and hard over the last few weeks I'd decided no more tube. After the nurse withdrew the tube, I told her that I didn't want her to insert another. I didn't want her to have any more tubes, I wanted to try and feed her myself. She looked at me with a puzzled look on her face and was clearly surprised at what I had said.

Moreover, with authority stamped in her voice she said that she didn't agree with me and that it was very important, for the moment at least, that Catherine was to be fed by the tube and said the tube was to remain. Nevertheless, I stood my ground.

After a mildly heated conversation, she said she would have to report me to the doctor and tell him that I had refused a feeding tube for my daughter.

I said "Ok that's just fine with me, but I want to you to understand that she's been getting fed by this method for such a long time now and I don't want anyone to start feeling complacent and to just carry on the same way without even trying something else! As far as I could see, Catherine wasn't making any improvements in the feeding department. I also felt that she never would if we didn't try. And furthermore she couldn't live the rest of her life being fed by a tube"

She said that she totally understood how I felt but, for now, it was the best way and the only way that Catherine could be fed; and if she didn't insert the tube now, how did I propose to feed her? I told her that I was going to try to feed her from a spoon. I was going to buy some Heinz baby dinners, the very first ones.

She shook her head and insisted that Catherine was to have the tube because she had to have nourishment. How could I argue with the nurse, she knew a great deal more than I regarding being tube feeding. So, I relented for the time being. I sat and held Catherine's hand and watched as the nurse inserted the tube.

Before she left I said that I understood her anxieties about Catherine, but I had mine as well. I just wanted to try and if it didn't work out then I'd have no objection to the feeding tube. After all I didn't want my child to be hungry least of all put her in any danger.

She replied that she would have a word with my doctor and relay my anxieties to him regarding the feeding tube. I knew my doctor would understand because he had always supported me; but I also knew that this would be different.

A couple of days later when the nurse came to change Catherine's tube she said that she had spoken to my doctor and he had said. The oesophageal tube was the only way to give Catherine all the nutrients and vitamins she needed. Therefore, for now we must use it, unless we see any signs that would tell us anything different. So there it was—I had my answer, but I wasn't going to give up. As the weeks went by the nurse and I would talk about the tube and of me wanting to try to feed her myself.

One morning she said that she had been thinking about how I wanted to feed Catherine myself; and suggested that while she was there the following morning we could try some baby dinner from a spoon. I was thrilled when she said that. I even kissed her on the cheek. She just laughed and said see you in the morning.

As soon as she'd gone I put Catherine in the wheelchair and walked to the shops. I went straight to the chemist and I bought six tins of Heinz first baby dinners because they were just like paste. I hardly slept that night I was so excited and eager and I could hardly wait for the morning to come. I desperately wanted to get rid of that awful tube.

Before the nurse came I half filled a small sauce-pan with boiling water, then after lowering the heat I placed a tin of first baby dinner into the simmering water so it would be just right; hopefully just right to feed Catherine with.

When the nurse came, I told her that I had prepared the baby dinner. She smiled and nodded her head and went into the front room where Catherine sat washed, dressed and propped up with cushions waiting for her. Slowly and carefully, she extracted the tube, as she did every other day. She cleaned the plaster mark that the tape had left on Catherine's cheek, which had secured the tube and checked her temperature. I went into the kitchen, opened the tiny tin, and placed it on to a warm cereal bowl. I thought this was it!

I placed a large tea-towel over Catherine's chest and sat on the couch beside her. The nurse said, "Ok if you feel ready you can try now." She sat on a chair opposite and watched me.

Before I began, I showed Catherine the bowl and I told her what I was going to do. I put a small amount of the food on a teaspoon and very carefully placed it onto her tongue; there was no response— it just stayed there. Then the liquid started to dribble down the side of her chin so I pushed it back gently into her mouth. There was a slight movement at the side of her mouth and her hand moved slowly. I thought just for one fleeting moment that she was trying to bring her hand up toward her mouth. I felt that she was trying to react and my heart began beating anxiously. I couldn't tell if she had swallowed some of the food because it just seemed to dribble out. I put another tiny amount in her mouth, all the time I kept talking to her telling her what was happening. The nurse kept watching. I kept placing a half-teaspoon of food onto her tongue. I was certain that some of it was finding its way into her stomach but I wasn't sure. I kept looking at her throat hoping for a swallowing reflex but I couldn't see one, but I kept on trying.

After about half an hour the nurse said, "I don't think that any food, well as much as she would need, has reached her stomach; but you could try again in a day or so when I'm back on duty. I'll have to insert her tube now she has to be nourished." Needless to say, I felt a bit let down but at least I was allowed to try. I was going to try again but only while Catherine's regular nurse was there because sometimes throughout the week it could be a different nurse. So again a couple of days later I followed the same procedure and did so for the next few weeks.

Until one day the nurse and I saw a swallowing reflection from her throat, we looked at each other and smiled. I carried on and bit by bit she managed to swallow some food but I also noticed her tongue didn't seem able to move!

As time went on Catherine began to progress with spoon feeding so much so she was able to manage about half a tin.

Because there was always a mess while I was trying to feed her, I'd have to cover her chest with a small hand towel before I began. Nevertheless, I was made up and I think the nurse was as well because she'd just look at Catherine and say, "Well done Catherine," and pat me on the shoulder on her way out.

During the following couple of months, we removed the tube completely because she was able to have a full tin of baby food twice a day plus a baby pudding. I must say she was still dribbling and making a mess but at least she was having about three quarters of a dinner and a pudding twice a day.

So I decided to make an eating plan. For breakfast each day, I mixed up a small bowl of Complan and fed it to Catherine on a teaspoon. Then at lunchtime and teatime, I'd give her a baby first dinner and baby pudding. Slowly but surely and day by day, she was beginning to get stronger and more alert. Her father and I and her family of course, were delighted, but in the back of my mind, I kept wondering why she didn't move her mouth or her tongue.

On reflection, I could understand at the time if the nurse had felt that I was putting her under pressure but I wasn't. It's because I didn't want to just accept that the tube was the only way or how long it was going to go on for; surely she couldn't live the rest of her life being fed by this method.

I knew that I wouldn't be successful at first but I had just wanted to try.

Without the help and support from the district nurse I don't think, in fact I knew that I would never have been able to do it by myself.

Over the following months, the visits from the nurse became less and less because Catherine didn't have to have the tube anymore; but she would call in once or twice just to check that all was well.

The next thing was I going to try to give Catherine some fluid. I began by putting a small quantity of water into a glass and drop-by-drop from the spoon; I'd placed the water onto her tongue. Sometimes she would cough and I'd panic because I was scared stiff of her choking. Each time she coughed, I'd wait a while and try again.

A couple of days later while I was shopping I bought a large Jaffa orange. I was going to try a different taste than just water; little did I know at that time that she couldn't taste anything. I squeezed the Jaffa orange and got about an ounce and a half of pure orange juice, then, drop-by-drop from the spoon; I put it onto her tongue. I know that she wouldn't be able to have it all, because some of the juice would trickled down the side of her mouth; but I did think some of it managed to trickle down her throat as well. If she coughed, which she did most of the time as I was trying to feed her, I would stop right away. Then I would smile at her and tell her that everything was alright and she was doing just fine. I always had to place a towel under her chin to try to minimize the wetness on her chest; but every day I kept trying

DURING THOSE weeks, when I was beginning to have some success with the Heinz first baby dinners, one of my friends had written to Heinz Foods. She explained about Catherine and how I was trying to feed her Heinz baby first dinners with a spoon and that, in between Catherine was being tube fed.

I felt absolutely, bowled over, when a couple of weeks later a post office van drew up outside my house and the man passed me a small cardboard carton.

When I asked him what it was he said "According to the label on the carton love I think it's from a well-wisher"

As he drove off, I went back into the house and opened the carton. I couldn't believe it. Heinz Foods had very kindly sent me two dozen first baby dinners and two dozen baby puddings. I stood for a minute and just stared at the contents and thought how wonderful and kind of Heinz. There was also a letter enclosed that wished me well and said that they would be delighted if and when I had the time to let them know how Catherine was progressing.

The following day after I fed her, I wrote to Heinz Foods and thanked them for their kindness and generosity, and yes, of course I will keep them informed of Catherine's progress.

Day after day, I carried on doing the same thing and day-by-day she seemed to becoming more aware. The district nurse was delighted with her progress.

She told the doctor about what I was trying to do. He came out to see her and was pleased to see really, positive progress. He told me to carry on the good work and he would call in to see her again. Even though she was so badly handicapped, her responses were very encouraging.

As time went on, I started to get a bit more adventurous. I mixed some packet mash potato because the texture was smoother. I could still only use a small spoon because I had to be very cautious I didn't want her to choke. I bought the biggest baby bibs that I could find to cover her chest to protect it from the constant slobbering.

Her father and I were due to take her back to the hospital for an assessment very soon. The main question we wanted to ask was why there were no signs of speech.

Every evening after tea the ice cream man would come around, ringing his bell, summer, autumn, winter or spring. It didn't matter about the weather, he called every evening. One particular evening I bought four ice cream cornets instead of three. I was going to try Catherine with an ice cream. First, I showed her the ice cream cornet then I put the cornet in her hand and I brought it up to her mouth. I spread the ice cream onto her lips and pushed a bit onto her tongue, but there was no movement from her tongue. Her father and I were puzzled. Couldn't she taste the ice cream? Why didn't she put her tongue out?

However, what happened next perked us up. While she was still holding the ice cream cornet that was beginning to melt and dribbling onto her dress, she was actually trying to bring it up to her mouth herself, but she missed her mouth and touched her cheek and her ear instead. That simple task that she had done was just wonderful because we knew that every single movement she made was a message sent by her brain. She wanted the ice cream cornet and knew she would have to bring it to her mouth so she could eat it and missed. The main thing was that she KNEW!

As I threw the melting ice cream into the bin, I thought what a great achievement. I couldn't wait to tell the nurse when she called in during her rounds. I knew that she would be delighted. We could hardly wait for the ice-cream man to call the next night so we could try again.

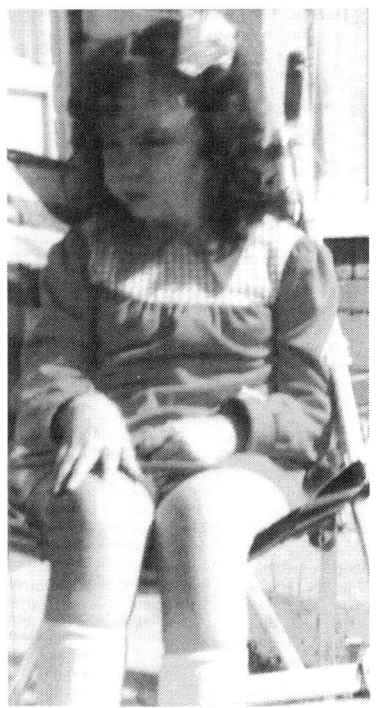

Catherine, age seven, enjoying the sunshine

10

One Step at a Time

CATHERINE'S PHYSIOTHERAPY sessions were doing her good and her limbs were suppler. Her father and I had to do some physiotherapy with her at home. Sometimes in the evening, he'd massage her legs with olive oil then place her against the living room wall and try to encourage her to walk to him. The children and I would hold our breath hoping against all hope that she would walk toward him but she couldn't; she'd slide down the living room wall and onto the floor. I was always anxious when this happened because the femur in her leg had been broken in the accident and it wasn't very strong.

The physiotherapy department at the hospital had lent us what they called a lobster pot. It was a small round steel frame with a canvas seat and in the middle; there were two holes in the seat for her legs to fit through. Her father or I would lift her up and sit her inside so that her feet were touching the floor. Even though she couldn't walk or talk she could push herself up and down the hall; it was great to see her like this because she looked so funny and seemed to enjoy what she was doing. Christine, Tony and Julianne were tickled pink to see her like that. Her father and I were made up with the progress she'd made but still there were no signs of speech.

In the meantime a neighbour who lived just a few doors down from us; told us that she was leaving and suggested that maybe we would like apply to the Housing Department to see if they would allow us to move in. Her house had a large through living room that would be ideal for us, and there was plenty of room for Catherine to move about in her lobster pot.

The new house had a telephone, which meant we wouldn't need to use the phone box on the corner of the road.

The following day her father made an appointment to see the manager at the housing department, to tell him about Catherine and the accident and how she was now progressing. The manager said he remembered hearing about a terrible accident Western Avenue where a little girl was badly injured, but that was some time ago. Her father said, "Yes it was his little girl who had been injured and she was the one they were discussing."

After hearing this, the manager said he was very understanding and sympathetic to our needs. But he said that he would have come to see her for himself and it would have to be this very week because he was going on holiday very soon. I thanked God we'd caught him before he left.

When he visited, he watched Catherine trying to get around in her lobster pot. He could also see we had three other children who were growing up fast and said with a big broad smile on his face, and much to our relief, that we could move into the bigger house but we were to wait until we received our letter of confirmation. True to his promise we received our letter of confirmation by hand a couple of days later.

We were so happy. The larger house would make such a difference. Our neighbour was absolutely delighted when we told her that we'd received confirmation and that we could move in as soon as she moved out. She said that when she'd decided to move house she thought of us and knew that we only had a parlour house which restricted Catherine's manoeuvring in her lobster pot.

Just two weeks later, my neighbour moved out early morning and we moved in later on the same day. It was better for all of us and gave Catherine the room she needed to manoeuvre in her lobster pot.

Over the following months, Catherine's progress was slow but steady. Every four weeks the pick-up ambulance would call for her and I would take her to her appointment with the physio at the hospital.

I told physiotherapist that sometimes I thought Catherine was going to get out of the armchair and walk to me, because she would stand up, then just when we'd think she was about to take a step she'd sit down again. I just didn't think she felt confident enough.

She said that sounded wonderful and agreed that it was lack of confidence. Then she took hold of Catherine's hand and walked her very slowly around the room. There were safety bars for her to hold onto if she felt nervous. Then she stood her by the wall and stepped back a little, then, with big encouraging smile I asked her to walk to me. She took a couple of tottering steps then she panicked and I caught her before she fell. The physiotherapist and I clapped our hands and said, "Well done Catherine that was just wonderful"

I told the physiotherapist that I'd decided to leave the lobster pot behind because I didn't think she would need it anymore. I was going to walk Catherine very slowly to the entrance of the hospital, which were only a few yards. Then when the ambulance dropped us off at home, she only had a little path to walk to our front door.

She laughed and said, "No I don't think she needs it anymore and it won't be long before she gains her confidence" She walked with Catherine and I to the bench where we could sit and wait until the ambulance arrived.

When I got home I told her father, brother and sisters what had happened, and they were made up. They already knew she had been trying for a couple of weeks but she just wasn't confident enough.

Then low and behold the following night, after I had bathed her and put her pyjamas on I walked her downstairs with me walking in front of her. The council had placed a rail on the wall at the side of the stairs for her to hold onto.

We walked into the living room and I was holding her hand at all times. Then I placed her in the armchair by the window and went into the kitchen to put the kettle on. I was going to make some tea and toast for us both because there was only her and I in the house. I went back into the living room while I waited for the kettle to boil and sat in the other chair opposite to were Catherine was sitting. Then what happened next and to my amazement, she stood up and began to walk toward me. My heart was beating so fast I thought it was going to burst out of my chest. Was I imagining she was walking to me—wobbly—but walking? I couldn't speak. I just took her hand and placed her back gently onto the chair, then I kissed her hand, looked into her face and said. "Well done my clever girl" I returned to my chair and smiled at her. Then she stood up and walked to me again. I held her tight and kissed her. What an achievement! This was so fantastic; our lovely girl was able to walk again.

In the meantime, the kettle was whistling like mad. I ran into the kitchen took the kettle off and opened the back door to let the steam out. I could hardly wait until everyone came home. Her father, brother Tony and sisters Christine and Julianne, were overjoyed and absolutely delighted to know that their little sister was slowly but surely getting stronger.

Yes, Catherine being able to walk again had brought such a lot of happiness to us and hope for her future!

At home she began to feel more confident and would walk from the living room into the kitchen, but I also noticed that she walked with a notable gait. She wasn't confident enough to walk outside just yet, but

I knew that would come.

Because she had begun to walk again I decided that the next thing I would try would be to try toilet train her. She had to use a commode which was alright for Catherine but not very pleasant for my other children.

Also, I didn't want to carry on inserting suppositories and I know she didn't either, but she had to have help with her bowel movement and it wasn't very nice for either of us so the best thing for me to do was to try to toilet train her.

The first week was the worst, trying to explain to her what I wanted her to do and why. Each time I needed the toilet I would take her up to the bathroom with me and show her what I was doing. After a couple of weeks she caught on and begun to wee on the toilet. During these times I'd place a pad onto her panties which I hoped would slowly but surely eliminate the nappies. Sometimes there'd be an accident and I still had to insert suppositories until she was able to eat more solid food, but what could I expect—she had done so well and we were half way there

One day, a couple of weeks after Catherine had begun to walk I decided to take her for a walk to our local shops. As we walked I heard running footsteps behind me, as I turned a young woman stopped and smiled at me; then she nodded her head toward Catherine and said breathlessly "How's she doing"? "Well as you can see, I said proudly she's doing very well, just got to take it day by day"

What she said next was so unexpected. "You said she can't speak and I've just seen you talking to her"

I couldn't believe my ears and replied angrily "No she can't speak and another thing it's a bloody good job that you're not her mother; because you would properly sit her on a stool in the corner of your living room place a dunces hat on her head and when someone calls to see you would say to them just ignore her because she can't speak, now go away from me you stupid ignorant woman." She didn't answer me; she just gave me a terrible look and walked quickly away. I looked at Catherine and said "God help us Catherine there's some really stupid people about" she looked up at me and smiled then we walked on. A week later after that incident, my daughter Christine was going to the post office, which was just down the road, and she took Catherine with her. Unfortunately while they were waiting to be served Catherine fell to the floor and began fitting; Christine knelt down beside her and kept talking to her until she came out of it. Then a few minutes later, when she felt that Catherine was alright, she took her hand and walked slowly back home. I was appalled and angry when Christine had told me what had happened and though-out her ordeal not one person offered to help or comfort her. Once again the head of ignorance had raised its ugly head.

~ 11 ~

Hadn't She Suffered Enough

AS WE sat in the waiting room, Catherine's father and I went over the questions that we were going to ask the doctor. Our main concerns were although Catherine was making steady progress, such as, not only had I been successful feeding her from a spoon, the oesophageal tube was finished with and she was able to sit at the table with her family. But I'd noticed that when I'd place a large spoon in her right hand and try to encourage her to scoop some food from her plate and onto her spoon she'd try to bring the spoon up to her mouth without success and the food would fall off. If I went to straighten her arm, she would pull it away.

We also noticed that when she smiled her mouth looked lopsided. Sometimes she would slobber just like a baby, so much so, I'd bought some toddler plastic pinafores to cover her with to protect her chest. And, could he also tell us why there were no signs of speech?

Another break through (well we thought it was) since we'd moved into the bigger house she was being more active and he could see she was able to walk. We knew that she had broken her femur in her left leg during the accident but recently it looked as if she was walking knock kneed.

Another observation was she began to move her eyes to one side, as if she was watching someone but there was nobody there.

When we put these comments to him, his reply was devastating.

He said, "The results of Catherine's injuries were beginning to show themselves, and all of her symptoms bore the hallmark of a person who had suffered a stroke! And yes, while Catherine had made good progress throughout the last year, it was too early to say how her progress would continue because the results of her injuries would become more visible as time went on. Also you must try and take note of how many times she moves her eyes to the side, for instance, is it happening more often? Does it happen more on one day and lesser the next? But it doesn't really matter what time of day"

He widened his eyes, pursed his lips and with nod of his head said,

"Mmm ok then, I will see Catherine in three months time. An appointment will be sent out to you"

Her father and I looked at one another in disbelief. How could that be? He must be wrong. Catherine was only a little girl; only old people suffered strokes. But the doctor was adamant in his diagnosis. Catherine had suffered a stroke when she had had the accident and all the signs were there to prove it. I felt as if I had suffered a severe punch in the stomach and by the look on her father's face, he felt the same. So we came away feeling absolutely devastated. We never expected to hear any of that, we were just hoping for some answers but sadly, they weren't the ones that we had hoped for. Before her next appointment, which was in three months time we found out what the movement in her eyes were.

One morning, a week or so after we'd seen the doctor at the hospital, I noticed to my horror, that when she moved her eyes this time she closed them before falling onto the living room floor; her little body shaking violently. I knelt on the floor beside her and called her name. Eventually she opened her eyes but she was very drowsy. As I held her close to me, she felt like a rag doll.

I lifted her up, placed her gently on the couch, and ran upstairs for a blanket to cover her. I rang my doctor and told him what had happened and he came out to see her after his morning surgery. He told me that unfortunately she had suffered an epileptic fit, which was evidence of a brain injury, which unfortunately, was beginning to manifest. He said he was going to make an appointment for her to see a specialist at Walton Hospital.

As I stood watching her sleeping, tears began to run down my face. I just couldn't believe it, hadn't she suffered enough? Then I remembered what the doctor had said when I'd told him about when she moves her eyes as if she was watching someone but there was nobody there.

I told her father when he came home what had happened and he was just as upset as I was. I felt like we were walking backwards instead of forwards.

Looking for Support

ABOUT SIX weeks later Catherine's appointment came for Walton Hospital. She was to see someone who specialised in epilepsy.

I found it very easy to talk to the specialist. He said that he understood my anxieties over the epilepsy. Then he began to explain why Catherine had begun to have fits.

The reason was because of the terrible injures she had received to her brain at the time of the accident. That even though there weren't any warning signs at first they can come later; for example, when she'd began to move her eyes and looked to the side.

He said that Catherine had Petit Mal a form of epilepsy. He made out a prescription for some medication for her called Epinutem and said he'd like to see her again in three months time. An appointment would be sent through the post. I went to the chemist as soon as I got home and picked up the prescription. It wasn't in tablet form; it was a thick pink liquid.

Later that evening when everyone had gone to bed, I began to fear that things looked as if they were getting worse for Catherine instead of better. All kinds of questions were running through my troubled mind. What were we to do? Where was I to go from here? Who do I turn to? Surely, there must be someone to help us.

I decided to make an appointment to see my doctor; he was always very supportive and understanding. He said that he would get in touch with someone from our local health centre that may be able to help and advise me.

A couple of days later I received a phone call from a health visitor. She was going to come out to see how I was coping.

When she came, I told her that I was beginning to feel very anxious about leaving Catherine on her own. Like when I have to put washing out or go upstairs to the toilet, or when I was in the kitchen, just in case she had a fit and banged her head. I also told her that with no one to talk to about it I was beginning to feel isolated. She listened to all I had to say and totally understood why I was so worried. She tried to reassure me that there were many people who suffered from epilepsy and with the right medication; some people were able to lead constructive lives.

Before she left she gave me a number to ring for the social services and said they may be able to help and advice me.

After she left, I rang the number and a young man answered. He was very pleasant to talk to and reassured me that he will call and see me in the very near future.

Just a few days later, he came to see us. After we'd introduced ourselves and made some small talk he asked me all about Catherine's accident; what her injuries were and what progress she had made. Then he asked me to tell him about my own anxieties and about my concerns for Catherine's future. As I spoke, he took notes. I told him that she couldn't speak and she had begun to have fits called Petite Mal, not knowing at the time that the fits were going to get worse. I also told him that I felt that she needed some kind of stimulation because she was just sitting in house with me every day.

The only outing we had was a walk to the local shops and back and then I'd have to put her in her wheelchair because she wasn't confident to walk outside yet.

After chatting for a while, he suggested that I let Catherine go to a small centre in Garston, which provides some facilities for mentally handicapped children and where she would mix with other children who were just like her. He told me there were other children at the centre who had epilepsy and far as he knows, they go to the swimming baths once a week. He advised me not to worry about Catherine because the staff at the centre were a small group of very caring professionals. He said a bus would pick Catherine up each morning at 9 and return her at 3:30. The driver would have an escort to ensure the children's safety. Then he asked me what I thought. I looked at Catherine and she smiled. I said it sounded just what she and I needed. He then said he would speak to the person in charge of the centre and see if they could fit Catherine in and he would ring me the next day.

As I closed the front door behind him, I heard a thud. Catherine was lying on the living room floor shaking she was having a fit. I knelt down beside her and kept talking to her as I always did until she eventually came around.

Later the following afternoon, the man who had come to see me about Catherine going to the centre in Garston rang me. Assigned as Catherine's social worker he arranged to meet us at the centre the following day so we could look around the facility and meet the staff.

He also said that he had managed to get Catherine an appointment with a speech therapist who would visit Catherine at the centre when she took up her place.

I was made up to hear this and looking forward to meeting them. At last, something good was happening for her.

As Catherine and I walked into the day centre hand in hand, a lady came towards us with a beautiful smile and introduced herself as the manager. She said that she had heard all about Catherine and had been looking forward to meeting her.

As we walked around the centre, she explained all that was going on and what their aim for these special children were. I was very impressed. It was only small but it had a lovely warm friendly atmosphere. The staff we met were friendly and spoke to Catherine like they had known her for a long time. After the walk-about, we went into the office and had a cup of tea. By the time we left, all was decided; Catherine was to start at the centre after the Easter holidays. I felt so happy this was just what Catherine needed. It was 1974

Every morning at 9:30 a dark blue mini bus would call for Catherine, take her to the centre in Garston, and return at 3-30 in the afternoon. The driver and the escort were really nice people and as time went by they and Catherine got to know one another. She seemed to be enjoying her time there and we received some favourable reports from the staff. They also sent me some lovely photographs of her that they had taken.

One photograph was taken while she was making cakes with some of the children; another was in the swimming baths wearing armbands of course, and being supported by two of the staff. There was also a photograph of when she was having a screaming fit and clapping her hands angrily, which I'd noticed seemed to be happening more frequently. When this happened, I knew it must have been frustration from lack of speech.

Unfortunately, over the following months she had a couple of terrible fits where she begun foaming at the mouth. I rang my doctor and told him about what was happening; he asked me when her next appointment at the hospital to see the specialist was? I told him in about six week's time. He said that we were to wait for that appointment because there was nothing he could do until Catherine saw the specialist.

The six weeks went by slowly as we waited for our appointment to see the specialist. At last the day came. I told him Catherine had been foaming at the mouth during her last four or five fits. Then after she'd come round her eyes would be glazed, she would be very tired and sleep for a couple of hours, we were very worried about her. And I'd also noticed that her gums where beginning to swell.

He said unfortunately, the Petite Mal had progressed into full epilepsy and she was having Grand Mal fits. This meant that he would have to change Catherine's medication. I replied that I was so glad to hear of the medication change because I didn't think (in fact I knew) the Epinutem wasn't doing her any good because her fits were getting worse and it was making her gums swell.

The new prescription was for Epilim and I hoped it would bring Catherine's fits under control.

Before I left, he said I was to bring her back in four months time which would hopefully give time for the new medication to get into her system. Armed with our new prescription I sat in the waiting room with Catherine and waited for the ambulance to take us home.

As soon as we got home we had a cup of tea, then I put Catherine in her wheel chair and went to the chemist to get her new medication. I gave her the first one before she went to bed and one in the morning as prescribed.

And so we carried on and Catherine went on the bus to the little centre as usual. I knew she was alright there because the staff looked after her so well and if they were worried they would ring me. We had to carry on as normal as we had our other three children to take care of. It must have been awful for them to see their little sister suffer from those horrible fits. Sometimes a couple of weeks could go by without any fits, but then she could have two in one day; you just couldn't predict when they would attack.

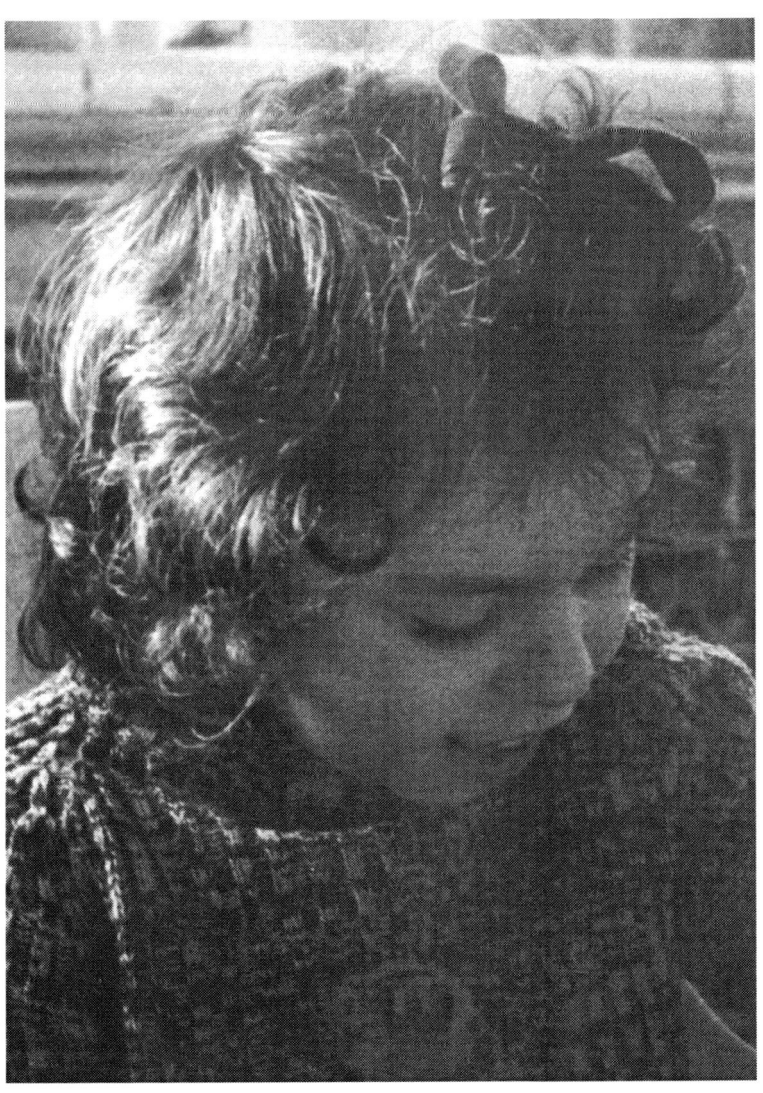

Catherine, age nine

~ 13 ~

Shattered

I WAS devastated at the news that Catherine's fits had turned into full-blown epilepsy because on top of that, just a few months earlier, we'd been told that Catherine had suffered a stroke due to the road accident. I tried to speak to her father about it but all he said was "Just leave it for now. Enough!" then he put on his coat and went out.

At the same time, my son Tony came running down the stairs and shouted to me "I'm going out Mum. I'll see you after" I heard the front door shut behind him.

My eldest daughter Christine was in the front room with her friend; they were singing along to "Ride a White Swan" a Marc Bolan record; her idol at the time.

My daughter Julianne, Catherine and I were watching TV.

I couldn't concentrate. I was beginning to feel as if I were in an abyss. After all she'd achieved and now this. Her father was also giving me cause for concern. He was going out more and more and wouldn't come back till the children had gone to bed. I think he was beginning to find the constant bad news hard to cope with, but then so did I. We were supposed to be in this together; Catherine needed both of us. I just felt like just crawling away to hide somewhere—anywhere, away from the constant torment.

One evening when the children had gone out to meet their friends, Catherine, her father and I were alone and it gave me the opportunity to try speaking to him.

I said "I know you're finding it hard to cope and believe me so am I, but you must look at it this way. Catherine has her age on her side, she's only eight and a half -years -old and she's making progress, no matter how slow, it is happening. Just look at what she's done in such a short time. She's eating at the table with us, she's walking, she's toilet trained, and hopefully the medication will sort the epilepsy out". This pep talk would help him, but only for a short time because he would slip right back into his depression again.

He would look at her with eyes full of tears and say "Why did God do this to her? She's never, ever, going to be able to look after herself, is she?"

Our marriage was being destroyed by the constant stress and my poor children were suffering too. Seeing their little sister injured and in constant need of my attention must have been awful for them. Catherine's accident was the worst thing that had ever happen to us; little did we know that there was more to come.

It was the morning of November 25th 1975. Tony and Julianne had left for school. The special bus had called at 9 -30 to pick Catherine up and take her to her day centre until half three. She was walking badly but, she was walking

Christine, our eldest daughter, had started work in a newly opened clothing store in a nearby shopping centre. She seemed to have grown up so fast. She was a proper little lady and an excellent support for me; her father and I were very proud of her. She also had a boyfriend who worked at a local bakery.

This was the day I was going to visit my paternal grandmother who was very ill. She lived with my aunty Mary and her husband in Croxteth, in the north of Liverpool. Before I left the house, I ran up the stairs and popped my head around my husband's bedroom door. He was lying on his side facing the bedroom window.

I told him where I was going and that I would be back before the children came home. He didn't answer me, but there was nothing strange about that. Sadly, we were like two ships that sailed through the night—romance was not even on our radar. I left the house and walked quickly to the bus stop. I had to get two buses and I hurried, not wanting to miss the connection because one bus only ran every half-hour.

I loved my Nan and aunty Mary very much because, they were always so good to my children and me. They had supported me throughout some of my most trying times. After spending a couple of hours with them it was time to leave. I didn't have to wait long for the first bus and made my second connection on time. I had to get some shopping before I went home, so instead of getting off the bus at my usual stop I carried on to the main shopping centre. After buying a few groceries, I still had some time before the children were due in from school so I did the fifteen-minute walk home.

As I drew near to where I lived, I could see the back of my house and noticed that the curtains in my husband's bedroom were still drawn. I thought that was strange because no matter the weather we always had the windows opened.

I quickened my step and turned the corner; mine was the second house. I hurried down the path, put my key in the lock and opened the front door. Christine's boyfriend Keith, had just come in from work and was in the kitchen making a cup of tea. He'd had a motorbike accident and I'd given him permission to stay with us so he could attend the hospital and wouldn't lose any time off work. At the time, he lived with his family in Runcorn but he worked at a major bakery nearby. I asked him if my husband had gone out. He said he didn't know because he'd only come in a couple of minutes before me.

I ran upstairs and noticed that the bedroom door was still ajar, the same way as it was when I left it that morning and the room looked very dark. I thought my husband must have gone out and forgotten to open the curtains. I pushed open the bedroom door and walked around the bed to the window. As I turned around, I saw that Tony was lying in the same position, as he was when I'd left that morning. I immediately knew there was something wrong. I went over to him and gently spoke his name, then I touched his forehead with my fingertips and to my horror, he felt cold, so very very cold.

I ran down the stairs screaming for Keith to get an ambulance. I opened the front door and ran out onto the street. I knocked on my neighbour's door but there was no answer. I ran back into the house. This wasn't really happening. I would wake in a few moments out of this nightmare.

Keith said that the ambulance was on its way. He also rang for my daughter Christine to come home. I asked him to ring for my aunty Annie because I needed her and she didn't live too far away. While we were waiting for the ambulance to arrive, I paced up and down the hall, repeating over, and over again, "He can't be dead! He can't be dead!"

Within a couple of minutes, which seemed like an hour, an ambulance pulled up outside the house and a police car screeched to a halt at the same time.

The ambulance men ran upstairs and were there for such a long time. Then, after what seemed like an eternity they brought Tony downstairs on a stretcher then placed him in the ambulance and I clambered in behind. I placed my hand on his forehead but he didn't move; he just looked as if he was fast asleep. I looked at the ambulance man who was with me in the back of the ambulance and said, "He's dead isn't he?" He looked at me kindly and replied "Wait until we get to the hospital sweetheart they'll be able to tell you all you need to know."

When we arrived at the hospital, the ambulance men took Tony away and a police officer asked me to accompany him. A nurse showed us both into a doctor's office, which she said, would be vacant for a little while.

He spoke to me gently and said, "I've just got to ask you a couple of questions." I nodded my head and said, "Ok." He asked me, what time I had left the house. Where had I been and what time did I get back? As I spoke, he was writing it all down. While we were speaking, a nurse brought me a cup of tea and a sympathetic smile.

A short time later, I don't remember how long, a doctor came into the room. I knew by the look on his face that it was bad news. He said, "I'm so very sorry my dear your husband is dead; he was dead on arrival."

I stared at the doctor in disbelief. He said Tony was DEAD! DEAD! What a horrible word. It's final. It's finished. No more, hope. DEAD! Even though I knew deep down it was true, remembering how I had touched him and he was so cold, I still found it hard to accept. This was devastating news. He was only 39 years-old.

Then I began to panic. I had to get home to my children—they'd be waiting for me wanting to know what had happened. The police officer was very kind and said he would take me home straight away. On my way home I was thinking, what am I going to tell my children and how am I going to explain to them that their father is dead.

When I got home, my Aunty Annie was waiting for me. Keith was upstairs with Christine. She was very upset. My son Tony was in his room very distressed. I sat on his bed and tried to speak to him but he was inconsolable. Julianne was downstairs with my aunty Annie, and Catherine was sitting on the couch looking around at everyone. I didn't know which way to turn. I felt so lost and I began to shake.

Then my aunty Annie took hold of me and wrapped her arms about me saying "Oh my poor, poor girl." I hadn't felt that bad since that terrible day when we thought we were going to lose Catherine. This was a terrible shock for my children and I—their father was dead and it was so difficult to take in—so much tragedy in such a short time. I held my head in my hands and cried as I've never cried before.

IT WAS hard to figure out if Catherine understood what had happened, but having said that, the following day she had a terrible tantrum. She stamped her feet, clapped her hands furiously, and screamed. When eventually I'd managed to calm her down I sat her on the couch and looked into her face. I tried to explain to her what had happened and that everything was going to be just fine. I couldn't tell if she understood anything that I had said to her. After a little while she fell asleep, she was exhausted after being so upset. I lay her on the couch and covered her with a small blanket. I'd never seen her act that way before but it was the only way that she could express her feelings. There had been times she would be so frustrated that she would screech and clap her hands; but not as bad as what had just happened.

A couple of days later, a police officer came to see me. He said that I was to attend the Coroner's Court for a hearing. I didn't know what that meant and the police officer never explained. David, my brother-in-law was visiting me that day and said that he was going to come with me. I was glad about that because I didn't know where I was going or what I was going for.

When we arrived at the Coroner's Court, which was in Castle Street at the time, a police officer escorted me to a door on the right and told me to follow him up a flight of narrow stairs. David wasn't allowed to come with me. He would have to wait in the waiting room.

I was scared and upset. I didn't know what was happening because nobody had explained anything to me. When I got to the top of the stairs, I couldn't believe my eyes. I was standing in what looked like a witness box like the ones that you see in the films. As I looked around me, I noticed to my surprise and relief, my doctor was there. He smiled and nodded his head at me. I didn't know at that time that he and a couple of police officers were going to be witnesses.

I noticed to the left of me was a long desk with a high backed chair in the middle. There were people looking up at me and a police officer stood behind me. Then a voice boomed out that the Coroner had arrived; and then a man came out of a side door and sat on the high back chair. He looked at me and I stared back at him. He asked me my name and with a quivering voice, I told him.

Then he asked if I was the wife of the deceased and I answered yes, I was. Then he said the reason I'd been called to the Coroner's Court was because my husband had died at home and there would have to be a post-mortem. Then he went on to say there always had to be a post-mortem when a person dies at home; it was the law. He then said they would send for me again when the results of the post mortem were ready. I stared at him and nodded my head. Everything was happening so fast. I found it so hard to comprehend what was going on. I'd never been anywhere like that before—I certainly didn't know such places existed.

Then the police officer tapped me on the shoulder and I followed him downstairs to where David was waiting for me. "Come on love," David said gently, "let's get you home."

I was glad to get home. I was so tired of it all. My world had collapsed about me and I just couldn't take anymore. I'd had enough.

A couple of weeks later a police officer came to see me. He said that I had to attend the Coroner's Court again because the Coroner had received the results of the post-mortem. And, just like the last time, I stood in what looked like a witness box. As I looked about me, there were several people sitting in the allotted benches. My brother Michael, who had driven me to the court, explained to me that there were other people waiting for results of a post- mortem, people who just like me, had lost a loved one at home. My mother was sitting in the front row smiling up at me.

When the Coroner walked in everything went quiet; then he looked about the court and sat down on his high back chair. He looked at me and repeated what he asked me last time. Was I the wife of the deceased, I replied that I was. Then he opened the file in front of him and read out aloud the results of the post-mortem.

He said that the pathologist had found that my husband had died from Asphyxia; which meant that he'd choked on his own vomit. He'd been drinking and eating a lot the night he died and was drunk when he'd got into bed which was very dangerous. When he coughed in his sleep, the food had lodged in his windpipe and because of his alcohol intake, he was too drunk to spit it out and that's what killed him. Then the coroner looked at me and said that I could go and carry on with my arrangements.

As we left the Coroners Court, a man who introduced himself as the pathologist stopped me and asked if Tony had ever been abroad. I told him not to my knowledge. He said the reason he asked was that he had found that Tony's lungs were badly diseased. The only answer I could give him was that Tony had always had breathing problems and sometimes suffered from terrible asthmatic attacks; so much so, I would have to get an ambulance and he'd be taken to hospital. He nodded his head, thanked me, and seemed satisfied with what I had told him.

The following day after the Coroner told me I could make my arrangements for my husband's funeral; I rang the local funeral directors. The next day a representative from the funeral directors came to see me. He was very helpful and arranged everything for me; because I just didn't know what to do. As we talked I found it so very difficult and so strange talking about my husband in the past tense. Before he left, he reassured me that everything will be just fine and I wasn't to worry.

I didn't want my children to see their father being lowered into the ground. I wanted them to remember him just how he was.

On the day of the funeral, the weather was appalling; it rained constantly, it never stopped. As I walked to the plot where Tony was to rest, I was slipping and sliding in the mud. My brother took my arm and supported me as we walked between the graves.

I will never forget the scene of how, and when, they lowered Tony into his resting place. As I stared into the grave, the tears ran gently down my face as I remembered all that we'd been through; and all the time the rain made a gentle patter upon his coffin. It was so painful knowing where he was, and there was nothing I could do for him. The coroner could say what he liked because deep down I knew Tony had died from a broken heart.

My brother took my arm and guided me through the muddy ground to the waiting car.

When we arrived home people where coming in and out of the house. I wanted to shout, why don't you all go home. I just needed to be with my children. To this very day, I don't remember who was there. It was such a devastating time in my life.

~ 14 ~

Picking up the Pieces

TONY'S DEATH was another terrible blow that my children and I had to endure. Christmas came and went and we didn't care. However, I had to try to pull myself together. I had to show my children that we could be strong and we could carry on. After all, we had each other and by God's good grace that's exactly what we did.

Sadly, during the following months, there still didn't seem to be any improvement with the fits and it looked as if Epilem wasn't the answer. After expressing my anxieties with the specialist at her next appointment, he said that he would change Catherine's medication again. He tried her on a course of Tegretol, which thankfully after a couple of years, seemed to be controlling the fits, not completely of course, but it looked as if Tegretol was just the right for her.

Tony Junior and Julianne went back to school and the special bus came as usual to pick Catherine up to take her to the day centre and Christine returned to work. Sometimes it could be very difficult for her to get to work, she couldn't rely on the bus being on time, it only ran every half hour and that's if it turned up at all. Fed up with the saga of the bus Christine took the initiative and changed her job. She was a very sensible young woman for a sixteen-year-old and was so supportive and understanding of what had happened to us as a family. Maybe it was because of the circumstances she had witnessed in her young life that she had grown up much quicker

My one and only beloved son Tony, was also growing up fast. He was a very happy and affectionate young man with a mischievous smile and you just couldn't help but love him. At the time, he was struggling with becoming a teenager and would find fault with the most trivial things I said or did. I remember one time when he was acting rebellious with me and we were arguing. He said something hurtful to me then he ran out of the house and slammed the front door. As he ran down the street, I called after him but he didn't answer. As the evening drew on, I was beginning to get worried because there was no sign of him.

Then just after 10 o'clock, I heard a knock on the front door. When I answered the knock Tony was standing on the step and handed me something wrapped in paper. Then he smiled and said, "I'm sorry mum" When I opened the paper he'd bought me a fish from the chip van that used to be at the bottom of our road. I laughed and said, "Thanks, just what I wanted, I'm starving" and so we were friends again for the time being at least.

Sometimes, and without my knowledge, he'd slip small pieces of paper into my coat pocket that would say, "I love you" or "Best mum in the world" They always warmed my heart and at that time in my life they were such a comfort to me. Sometimes, when I found these special little notes I'd approach him and try to encourage him to talk about Catherine's accident, but he would brush it one side and refuse to talk about it. I went to see my doctor and told him how concerned I was about my son and how he'd refuse to talk about what happened. He said that Tony would talk about it when he was ready; but sadly, he never has, not to me anyway.

I know even today that he still has that picture in his mind of his little sister lying injured in the road. I know I do too and it's very painful. He and I know what a distressing picture that was on that terrible day on the 28th June 1972.

Julianne was growing up fast and had started her senior school just before her father had died. She was very outgoing and loved playing football on the field with the boys; sometimes they'd call for her to join the team if there was going to be a game; she was always bit of a tomboy. I remember one day some of the children that she'd been playing with came running over to the house; they told me that Julianne had fallen off the monkey ladder. I panicked and ran over to the field, she wasn't unconscious or anything but she was shaken. I put my arm about her waist and we walked quickly to the doctors, which was about a five or six minute walk from where we lived. After explaining to the receptionist what had happened she took us straight in to see the doctor. After he'd examined her thoroughly he said that as far as he could see she was fine, but if she showed any signs of drowsiness I was to get in touch with him. I was so relieved. Within a short while, she was herself again thank God!

It wasn't long before she let go of her tomboy image and begun to take an interest in her appearance.

My brother's wife Chris, who was a hairdresser at the time, gave her a new hairstyle. She looked so pretty and so grown up. Julianne was a brunette with a cast of auburn in her hair and dark brown eyes.

After having her head shaved after the accident, Catherine's hair had grown back from brown to dark brunette with a cast of auburn, and her eyes were speckled green and grey.

Christine was growing into beautiful tall blond with a strawberry cast in her hair and bright blue eyes.

Tony junior had light brown hair with a strawberry cast and his eyes were hazel just like mine. I was so lucky to have four beautiful children.

Watching how my three other children were getting on with their lives I decided to go to the education department in Sir Thomas Street in Liverpool. I wanted to ask if it were at all possible that Catherine could return to her old school. They told me gently but firmly it was impossible for her to return to her old school.

The reason they gave me was she would need special attention, which could not be provided because, they couldn't afford to pay for a specialist teacher. She had to stay where she was at the three day a week special school. They did suggest that I talk to the social services department to see if they could help me any further. I said I would certainly think about it. Deep down I knew they were right about not allowing Catherine to go back to her old school, but I had to try.

So she stayed at the special school for three days a week. In between times, a speech therapist had been to see Catherine couple of times and did some little tests with her. He'd place different objects on the table in front of her then ask her to pick or point out certain ones; she'd do very well and sometimes she'd get eight items right out of ten which was excellent. However, her concentration wasn't very good and she'd just get bored and would refuse to do any more when asked. The staff at the centre was lovely and very caring but still no one could tell me why she couldn't speak.

Throughout it all, I found it very hard to accept that she was handicapped; after all, I kept reminding myself, she wasn't born handicapped. She was a beautiful nine pounds-ten ounce baby girl whom I had given birth to at home. Sometimes, when I went to the education department or the hospital I had to pinch myself, was I really talking about Catherine, my funny mischievous little girl? Then reality would kick in and with a terrible pain in my heart I would realise that YES, it was her we were talking about. Even today, Forty years later I still find it so hard!

Although she was walking, it was with a very noticeable gait. She still couldn't speak, chew or eat with a knife and fork. Sometimes she'd have terrible tantrums, stamp her feet, and clap her hands in frustration. I kept looking for an alternative but there didn't seem to be any. There were no rehabilitation units in 1976 and if there were, nobody ever told me about them. Anyone who suffers any sort of brain injury today would have a better chance of a full recovery depending of course on how severe their injuries were, what with all the modern day life saving machines and special after care programmes there are.

Of an evening after tea, Christine would go and see her boyfriend Keith. Tony would go out with his friends and Julianne would be out with her friends, which just left Catherine and me on our own in the house.

Now and again, my good friend and neighbour Hilda would call and keep me company for a while. Sometimes an old friend would visit but, when my visitors had left and my children had gone to bed, I was on my own again.

Occasionally when Christine returned home after her date with Keith, she and I would talk. She'd tell me all about what had happened that day in work, or where she and Keith had been that evening.

My children were a comfort for me. Their need for me gave me the courage to carry on, but that wasn't going to last forever; because eventually they would make their own way in life. I couldn't expect them to sit in the house with me—I just wanted them to carry on as normal as possible.

The year after my husband died, Christine and Keith were married in the same church as her father and I. It was a very cold day in November and a fine mist hung about that was threatening to turn into fog. I'm pleased to say that their photographer turned up and took some lovely photographs of their wedding. We held the celebrations in the church hall. My brother Michael gave Christine away. I love my brother, but it would have been so wonderful if her father could have given her away but, it wasn't to be.

Then joy of all joys a few months later Christine gave birth to a son. Keith and I went with her to the hospital when she was in labour, but after a while, I had to leave and get back home. No sooner had I reached home than Keith rang me and said Christine had given birth to a son. I couldn't believe it, I was a grandmother, me a Grandmother! I placed Catherine in her buggy and dashed around to my mum and dad's. They only lived around the corner from me and I just couldn't wait to tell them the news. My dad took a bottle of scotch from the cupboard, and then he, my mum and I wet my grandson's head, their first great grandson. I couldn't wait for visiting time to come. I was so excited.

When I got the hospital, Christine and her newborn son were in a lovely little room of their own. As soon as she saw me she said, "Never again mum! Never again! It was awful; how did you do it four times?"

I laughed at her reaction and said. "We've all said that but, it won't be as bad with the next one."

"Oh no mum—I mean it, I won't be having any more."

I just laughed it off. Then my heart swelled with joy as I held my first grandchild in my arms for the very first time. He was beautiful and so handsome. I felt truly blessed with happiness at the special moment in my life.

~ 15 ~

Our Visit to Cambridge

ONE EVENING while mashing Catherine's food, I began to wonder to myself how long she would have to have her food mashed like this. Surely, there must be something or someone that could help her to eat and swallow food normally before she got any older. She was now nine years old. I decided to go and see my doctor to see if he could give me any help or advice. He said understood the worries and anxieties that I had and after talking for some time, he said that he would send a letter to a certain doctor at Cambridge Hospital and request an assessment on Catherine's condition. Before I left the surgery, he told me that I wasn't to build my hopes up, but I was used to that advice which didn't mean anything to me anymore.

A week or so later I began to watch for the postman. I was waiting and hoping that he would soon bring the letter with Catherine's appointment to go to Cambridge. Then one day, after I returned home from shopping there was a letter lying on the hall mat stamped with a Cambridge postmark. I picked it up and held it to my breast for a minute then I sat on the bottom of the stairs and I opened it. Great news, we had an appointment for her to see a neurologist at Cambridge Hospital. The little voice in my head kept saying don't build your hopes up but I shrugged it off. We had an appointment that's all that mattered.

That evening I rang my brother Michael, I told him about the appointment, and he was delighted. He said that he would come with me and drive us to Cambridge; my mother wanted to come with us as well. Financially it was going to be tough because there was a consultation fee and the cost of our accommodation. My brother said that he would approach his shop steward in work to see if they could help, which he did a couple of days later.

Michael told his shop steward why we were going to Cambridge and the appointment. He explained that I would have to pay for the consultation and we would have to stay overnight. It was expensive and I was only in receipt of a widow's mother allowance and getting family allowance for two of my children. A few days later, the shop steward came to see my brother; he told him that Transport and General Union would like to help me in my situation. They offered to pay the consultation fee plus the hotel bill for me, Catherine, my brother and my mother. This was great news for us. Their kindness was overwhelming and gratefully accepted.

We arranged everything for our trip to Cambridge. June, Michael's wife offered to look after my family for me while I was away. My brother and his wife June were always so supportive to me. Then the great day for our journey arrived, I was so excited. We were all praying that this man would be able to tell me why Catherine couldn't chew her food and couldn't speak. My brother, Catherine, my mother and I all piled into the car and set off to Cambridge.

On our arrival at the Cambridge Hospital, we made our way to the reception desk and told the young woman behind the desk who we were and to whom we had come to see. She smiled and said politely for us to take a seat in the waiting room until they called Catherine's name.

We didn't have to wait long because a young woman, who introduced herself as the neurologist secretary, came in and asked if I would bring Catherine along as the doctor was waiting in his office to meet her. My mother and my brother wished us luck and said that they would stay right there and wait for us to return. As we entered the doctor's office, he stood up from behind his desk and smiled at us both; then held his hand out to me and introduced himself.

After the formal introductions, he asked me all about Catherine's accident. I did my best to answer his questions. All the time I was speaking, he was looking at Catherine and the side of her face that was slightly crooked. After about thirty minutes chatting about what her injuries were and how she sustained them I told him what the doctor had told her father and I when she went for her assessment at Myrtle Street children's hospital in Liverpool some time ago. He didn't say anything he just smiled and nodded his head. Then he said that he needed to take some messages from her brain and hoped this would give him a clearer picture. Then he stood up and said, "So if you would like to come with me we can get started."

We followed him into a brightly lit room where there were some monitoring machines. He asked me to sit Catherine with her back to one of the machines; eventually and after some friendly persuasion, she sat. Once she had settled, the doctor placed some headphones over her ears. There were wires attached to the headphones with tiny probes that rested on a long paper graph. When he turned on the machine

Catherine began to get upset, there wasn't any noise from the machine only a gentle buzzing sound, but she didn't like the headphones on her ears. The doctor smiled and reassured me that she wasn't in any danger.

I calmed her down and spoke to her quietly then took my place behind a glass partition where she could see me and I prayed silently. The tiny probes started to make a pattern on the paper graph that came slowly out of the machine.

When he had taken enough readings, he tore the paper carefully from the graph. Then he removed the headphones from Catherine's head and gestured to me to come and get her. She wasn't very happy because she didn't understand what was happening. I kept wondering what he was going to say. Would he be able to tell me why Catherine couldn't speak? Would she ever be able to speak again? These were the questions that have haunted me ever since she'd come out of the coma. The doctor looked at me and said, "Let's go back to my office and look at our findings. I felt as if I was going to burst. I wanted to know what was on the graph. He walked behind his desk and placed the paper graph in front of him and I watched his face as he ran his eyes over it. Then, after what seemed like forever, he sat up straight in his chair and looked at me.

Apparently, he said, even though Catherine's injuries were so bad from the accident, the messages on the graph, recorded from her brain, were good. I was hanging on to every word he said. Then he came to the part that I was waiting for. He said that he couldn't possibly tell me if Catherine would ever speak again and he couldn't possibly commit himself by saying that she ever would. He said that he wished that he could've given me the news that I wanted so badly, but unfortunately he couldn't. Then he ended with the same old familiar phase, but you must never give up.

Once again my hopes were dashed.

He stood up from behind his desk and clasped my hand. I thought there was sadness in his eyes as he wished us both all the very best for the future.

I smiled politely and thanked him for his time then I took Catherine's hand and walked out of his office. My brother and my mother stood up quickly in anticipation as Catherine and I walked into the waiting room; but they could tell by the look on my face that the news wasn't good.

I told them what the doctor had said. My brother put his arm around my shoulders and said "Never mind girl, you never know, there still could be someone out there who may be able to help her."

My mother said. "That's right girl, there's always new things coming out and you never know in the near future there could be a way of helping her."

I know they meant well but I felt so let down and dejected. The four of us walked out of the grounds of the hospital and made our way back to the hotel where we were staying overnight. We left for home early the following morning, less happy than we were when we had first arrived.

After the disappointment at Cambridge days turned into weeks, weeks turned into months. All the time dark clouds were beginning to gather. Every time I looked at Catherine, seeds of doubt about her condition were starting to take root. Could the doctor who gave us her first assessment when she had come out of the coma be right? He said that she would never be able to do anything for herself. Had I been in denial all this time? I was finding it harder to cope.

In the mean time life for my family and I moved on.

My eldest daughter Christine had married and had a little son of her own, and she called him Antony after her father. It was so sad that her father didn't live to see him. I was delighted with my little grandson he was gorgeous.

My son Tony had left school and had started work at T J Hughes in London Road Liverpool. I bought him a new blue jacket. He looked so handsome and I was so proud of him. It wasn't long before he had a girlfriend at work. I must say it wasn't his first girlfriend. The very first girl that he brought home to meet me was when he was just about six years old. One afternoon when he came home from school, he had a little girl with him. He brought her into the kitchen where I was preparing our tea. As he introduced her to me, he pointed out that her hair was black, just like mine, and her name was Sheila, just like mine. I was tickled pink. He was so, serious as he compared his first love to me. (My mother always called me Sheila so there would be no confusion since her name was Julia, and our whole family followed suit.)

My other daughter Julianne was her happy out-going self—thank God! She always had a smile no matter what. I was very proud of my family as we carried on with our day-to-day lives.

~ 16 ~

The Value of Friendship

TIME WENT on and my children were growing and living their lives by going out with friends, making new friends, and doing the things that young people do. Most evenings after washing and changing Catherine ready for bed, I'd find myself sitting on my own. Sometimes I would read, or try to read but I couldn't concentrate because my mind was always wondering to what was going to happen in the future. Then, while tears ran gently down my face I would try to put it all at the back of my mind, but it was always there. Even though I had my children, I was very lonely.

Though the little day centre that Catherine attended three days a week was good and the staff very caring; over a matter of time, I began to feel that I just couldn't cope with the constant caring day after day. I had no one to help me; I was completely on my own. I rang the social worker and she came out to see me. After talking it through, she found a solution that she hoped would benefit Catherine and I. Eventually she suggested that Catherine could go residential throughout the week and come home at weekends. That meant that I could get a job, which also meant that I would be able to socialise with the outside world, and so we decided, I would try it.

One day while I was out shopping, I bumped into my old friend Sue. We used to have such fun together when we were teenagers going to the Dove and Olive which was a newly built pub where every weekend different pop groups would be playing; which was fantastic for us because there wasn't any entertainment for young people in Speke at that time.

Sue said that she'd heard about Catherine's accident and Tony's death and what a terrible tragedy that must have been for me and my family. She said she would have loved to come to see me and often wondered how I was coping.

I told her that things were going alright at the moment; but I felt there was no future for Catherine or myself; well at least I couldn't see any the way the situation was at the time.

She told me that the relationship with her son's father had ended, so she and I were two lonely women—then we just looked at one another and laughed heartily. She suggested that maybe we could go out together one evening, maybe the pictures, just like old times, anything to break the monotony. I said that I would love to but I couldn't because I had Julianne and Catherine to take care of.

She sighed and said, "Ah well never mind, I understand, but what about tomorrow night if I call in for a cup of tea and a chat."

"Oh yes that would be great" I said.

"Ok it's a date!" she laughed. "I'll see you tomorrow night."

I looked at her as she walked away, remembering the times when I would go with her, to visit her mother when she was in hospital.

The first time I met my friend Sue was when I started my very first job after leaving school at Howard Ford in Woolton, which made nylon stockings (Bear Brand) I was 15 years old. I trained as a seamer and she worked in what they called the Hot Legs section; that was where, once the stockings had left my department, they would go to hers and be sized.

Everyone had a target to work toward, which were 250 pairs of stockings in a tub in a limited amount of time. We would be paid 10/- shillings for each tub. That's fifty pence in today's money. If there were anything wrong with your work it could be (and sometimes would be), taken out of your following week's wage. There was a bright side to it all; we could buy our nylons for 1/6 per pair, seven and a half pence in today's money.

Depending on what my expenses were, like paying for my keep and paying for my new bike I bought to use for work, I would be able to buy two pairs.

Sue had been in a children's home since she was two years old and her two younger brothers followed suit. The reason being her mother had been in bad health for many years and was too ill to look after her young family. Sue's father couldn't cope on his own because he had no one to help him, so consequently Sue and her two little brothers spent their first tender years of life and into their early teenage years, in care. I went with Sue to the hospital to see her mum a couple of times. Sometimes she'd be allowed home for a little while and I'd go to see her. Sadly she died in 1969 and Sue was broken-hearted. Sues' mum was a very quiet and gently spoken woman.

Sue came out of the home in 1953 when she became eighteen. She went to live with her father and looked after him until his death. She only lived two roads away from me, so we saw one another in and out of work, but as time went by, we went our separate ways.

I told my eldest daughter Christine about meeting my old friend Sue and what we'd been talking about. She was thrilled for me and encouraged me to go out with her. When I told Sue, what my daughter had said she was delighted.

Sue and I began to go out together once a week; it was all we could afford. Sometimes we'd return to our old haunt, The Dove and Olive, a place that held many memories for me and where I first met my husband Tony. I could visualise him standing by the door of the bar when he lifted his pint glass to me and mimed "Hiya,"

Now and again, there would be a group appearing at the Dove and Olive but it was mostly disco music now. The film "Saturday Night Fever" was all the rage at the time.

One night Sue and I went to the British Legion, we went to see a group who was very popular at the time; I think they were called, "The Real Thing" they were fantastic. We really enjoyed ourselves and for just a short while, I could give my troubled mind a break from worry.

Just as we were leaving Sue's neighbour, Harry walked in. He looked surprised to see us and said, "What are you two doing here?" She told him that we'd come to see the group and we were just going home. He said that he'd arranged to meet his mate there because they were going into town. Just then, his mate came in and walked over to where we were sitting. Harry introduced him and said his name was Bill, Bill Donal.

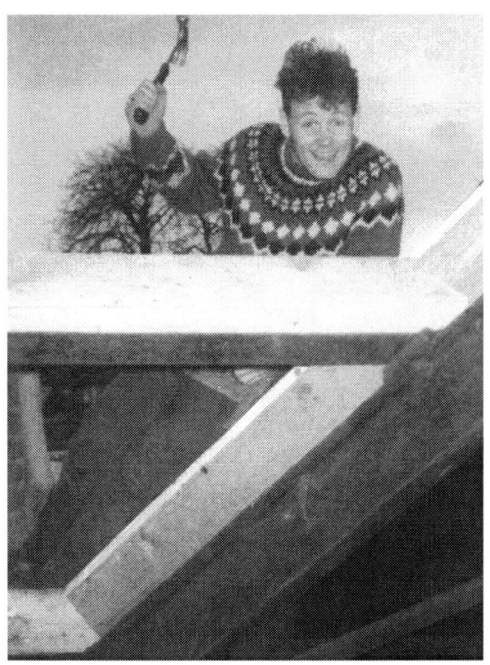

Catherine's brother, Tony at work

A Chance Meeting

IT WAS 1978 and getting near to Christmas; there was a lot to do and I had to get prepared. I had to get presents for my children and little grandson Antony. I wanted my children to have what they had always had, a great Christmas no matter how tough things had been.

One evening after tea, Sue came to see me. She said that she had bought two tickets for a New Years Eve party at the local parish church social club. I was so happy. It was something to look forward to, but the following day she came back and told me that the tickets she had bought were no good because we wouldn't be permitted into the entertainments room—they were for the bar only. She said when she went back to the club and asked if they would change the tickets, they were adamant and said that they couldn't because the entertainments room was full to capacity due to the amount of tickets that had been sold. That meant that we would have to sit in the bar all evening. We didn't want that, we wanted to be entertained. We weren't bothered about drinking because we only ever had a glass of wine each but we were so disappointed. Sue said that she would ask her neighbour Harry if he would be able to get us some tickets for the British Legion.

The next day she came to see me with a big smile on her face. She said as soon as she left me yesterday she went to see Harry and asked him about the tickets. He said that he would see what he could do because he was going to the British Legion later to meet his friend Bill after work. The following morning on his way to work Harry called and gave Sue two tickets. They were for two females, allocated only to members of the British Legion. Harry had given Sue his and Bill had given the other one for me if I wanted it.

We were thrilled now we could look forward to a good night out. My daughter Christine and her husband Keith offered to look after Julianne and Catherine for me. My son Tony was going out with his friends.

Harry suggested to Sue that it would be a good idea for us to get to the British Legion early so that we could get a good seat because

New Years Eve was a very special night and the place would be full to capacity.

When Sue and I arrived at the British Legion, there were two men on the door examining every ticket very carefully.

When it came to our turn, we confidently handed our tickets to the doorman. He gave us a big toothy grin and said "Alright girls go on in and enjoy yourselves!" Like two teenagers on their first night out, we walked into the entertainments room with our eyes wide open not knowing what to expect. The walls were decorated with colourful Christmas garlands, and on all the tables were party hats of different shapes and sizes. Everything looked so beautiful.

We managed to get ourselves a table so that our backs were against the wall and we'd be able see all that was going on. We both picked up a party hat from the table and put them on our heads then we looked at one another and went into pleats of laughter. Both of us were so happy and excited, we were going to enjoy ourselves and it was going to be a good night.

About an hour or so later Harry and his friend Bill, came into the hall looking round the crowded room for us. We both stood and waved to them and they waved back, came over, and joined us. After seeing that we were happy with our seating arrangements, they both went to the bar to get some drinks. I said I didn't want a drink. Bill looked at me smiled and said "You can't let the New Year in without drink now can you?"

I smiled back. "Ok just a small glass of wine then please." Just then the lights dimmed, the MC jumped up onto the stage and told a few jokes that weren't very funny but nobody cared because it was New Year's Eve. Then to a loud cheer, he introduced the act that was going to entertain us for the rest of the evening. The atmosphere was buzzing with excitement.

Sue and I got up to dance, but there wasn't much room on the dance floor which was jam packed because the group were very good; plus everyone was a bit tipsy. After a little while, Sue and I had to sit down because we were so out of breath.

Sue looked at her watch. It was five minutes to midnight, getting nearer to the bewitching hour. Bill and Harry jostled through the crowded room holding our drinks above their heads as they made their way back to our table.

Then MC jumped back onto the stage and everyone joined in as counted the seconds to till midnight, and then it came, "Happy New

Year everybody" he shouted at the top of his voice.

Everyone joined in and sang; "Auld Lang Syne" then hugged and kissed each other. Bill put his arms out to me and smiled. We kissed, hugged, and wished each other the very best for the future and Sue and Harry did the same. I hadn't felt so happy for such a long time. The atmosphere of the evening was wonderful and a New Year had begun.

When all the festivities were over at the British Legion, everyone began to make their way home. Bill said that his sister was having a New Years Eve party and asked would we like to go. I knew my family were alright because my daughter and her husband were looking after Catherine and Julianne. Sue was alright because her father would be there if her son Mark came home before her so we decide to go to the party. It was only a ten-minute walk from the British Legion to Bill's sister's house.

Bill introduced Sue and me to his sister Brenda, who welcomed us and offered us a New Year's drink inviting us to help ourselves at the buffet. As I looked around the room, a lovely warm feeling like a sense of belonging came over me. Like something, I hadn't felt since I was about six-years-old; when I met my father again when he came back from the war. I was only two years old when he left.

After about an hour I told Bill that I was going to make my way back home; I wanted to make sure that my family were alright. He got my coat for me and walked me home right to my front door. Before he left he asked would I like to go out with him the following Saturday? I said I would like to, but I had commitments at home and I couldn't promise anything, so we left it at that. That night as I lay in my bed I kept wondering what the hand of fate had in store for me this coming year.

About four or five weeks later Sue came to see me and asked if I would like to go out with her for a couple of hours the next Friday night because there was a band appearing at the British Legion who were very popular in the sixties. She said a night out would do us both good because since New Year's eve we had both felt a bit deflated.

When I told my daughter Christine, what Sue had said her reaction was, "You must go Mum! You go out with Sue and I'll be here for our Julianne and Cathy."

The following morning I went to see Sue and told her what Christine had said and she was made up, so we made our arrangements for next Friday night. We didn't need any female tickets this time!

We found ourselves a good seat right in the front of the stage so that we would have a good view of the group. I think they were The Moody Blues. They were fantastic and brought the house down. Sue and I really enjoyed ourselves.

Just as we were leaving someone called out to Sue, we both turned around, it was Harry. He asked how long we'd been there. We said that we'd been to see the group and we were just leaving. He said that he and Bill had just called in for a drink after work and they were just about to leave as well. Then Bill came out of the bar and looked surprised to see us, then after greeting each other with some small talk, it was decided that we'd all walk home together. When I reached my house, Bill asked me again if I would go out with him. I said that I couldn't possibly commit myself as I had responsibilities at home. His reply was that he would take a chance anyway and call on Saturday evening just in case I'd found a baby sitter.

My daughter Christine was tickled, pink when I told her what Bill had said and once again she encouraged me to go out and I must say it didn't take much encouragement. So, because of my daughter Christine and when my respite days were due, I was beginning to enjoy some sort of a life for myself no matter how limited.

Saturday evening came and so did Bill. I went outside when I saw his car drawing up outside my house. We chatted outside in the car for a while.

Then he said, he would like to see me again, would I go out with him next Tuesday evening. He said we could go to the Woolton Picture House to see John Travolta in Saturday night fever. I said yes, I'd like to. I'd already bought the record so it would be good to see the film, but once again I would have to see if Christine could baby sit for me. He said he would take a chance and call on Tuesday evening just in case, which he did. My daughter Christine once again looked after Catherine for me. She always encouraged me to go out and was happy to see that I was taking more care of myself.

So we began to see one another once a week and would sometimes make it a foursome with Sue and Harry. One evening when Bill called for me, it had been snowing, so he left his car outside my house and we walked to the British legion. We found a nice cosy corner where we could sit and chat. He asked me again would I consider us staying together as a couple, nothing heavy just go out together. I said that I would like that, but like I'd already told him I had commitments at home and it wasn't going to be easy because my family would have to come first. Then he looked at me, smiled, and said that he understood.

When we came out of the British Legion, it was bitterly cold and a fine film of ice shimmered over the ground. I wrapped my fake fur coat tightly about me and I put my arm through Bill's. He just smiled and said "Hold on tight love, the ground is treacherous"

It felt so right, so comfortable; it was as if we'd known one another for a life time. We had to walk slowly because the ground was like ice beneath our feet. We didn't bother with the bus, we walked, which gave me the opportunity to explain what my commitments were and to explain about Catherine. As we walked, I talked.

Of course, he knew that I was a widow; but he didn't know anything about Catherine. I told him everything about her. About the accident and all that, she had suffered; and of all the special needs that she would have for the rest of her life and she will always need to have someone to look after her. So because of this the social services advised me to let her go residential throughout the week and return home at weekends. The purpose was to give me a break and try to find some kind of life for myself in-between looking after my family. This meant I could get a job and this was all in hand. I held the fur collar of my coat around my ears because Jack Frost was beginning to bite at my fingers and toes. We stopped walking and Bill put his arms around me. His answer to all that I had told him was,

"All I can say is it must be very difficult for you but it won't make any difference to the way I feel about you, and I would still like us to continue to see each other every week"

I was so surprised. I didn't think that he'd felt that way about me because we hadn't known one another that long and I had been perfectly honest with him.

Just then as we stood talking on the corner, a couple of doors away from my front door, my son Tony walked by. He looked at us both, recognised me and gave me a terrible look, then, he walked into the house and slammed the front door. To say he wasn't pleased would be an understatement.

Bill and I decided to say goodnight, but before he left, he said that he would be calling for me next Saturday evening. I just said OK.

But deep down I thought, no he won't call on Saturday, he'll have had time to think properly about what I had told him about Catherine, and of course the disapproval of my son. It wasn't going to be easy and would be best to finish now before it gets serious.

During the week, my daughter Christine came to visit with my little grandson Antony. I told her of the conversation that Bill and I had had, also about Tony when he saw Bill and I together on the corner of the road.

She laughed and said, "You look better now than you've looked for a long time mum. If you're happy to be with Bill, stay with him. It's probably a bit of jealousy with our Tony. Just try it out with Bill and if it doesn't work out so be it, but I really would give it a try if I were you" I looked at her and thought wise words from one so young.

Saturday evening Bill's car pulled up outside my house. I was surprised to see him after what I had told him the other night. I went out to him and told him that I hadn't been expecting him. He smiled at me and said "Just put your coat on I need to speak to you I promise we won't be long. I went back into house where my daughter Julianne was sitting in living room with Catherine. Julianne was fifteen years old at the time and Tony had gone out. I asked her to look after Catherine and that I'd be just outside because Bill and I had something he wanted to talk about. She smiled and said, "That's ok mum"

Bill said that he'd been thinking about what I had told him about Catherine. He also said that he understood why Tony was angry and how he must have felt when he saw us on the corner even though we were only talking. He said that he'd tried to picture his own mother standing on the corner with a man and said that he would have probably felt the same. Nevertheless, we both knew that Tony was angry and upset.

Then he began to tell me about himself. His first job when he left school was at Milner's Safes where he worked for about twelve months, a job he hated. He said his father got him a job at Higsons brewery as second man on the bottle wagon and dray wagons. One day his boss suggested that it was time he went in for a driving test, which he did and was successful.

After some time when a vacancy came up for a driver's job on the wagons Bill got the job, which meant he would be out on the road making deliveries, plus the wages were better.

Sometime later Bill decided to go to Jersey in Channel Islands to work because some of his friends were already working there. They'd written to say there were lots labouring jobs on offer. So he gave in his notice and went to look for work in Jersey.

He got a job at the nurseries where they grew and nurtured some of the flowers for the Jersey Battle of Flowers. The nursery also grew tomatoes, some for seeding ready for the coming year. At Christmas,

Bill and his friends would come home to visit their families.

Because the job in Jersey was just seasonal work he decided to go back to the brewery in Liverpool and applied for work; luckily he got a job as a driver.

After working for the brewery for a couple of years he'd saved enough money to pay for his accommodation when he returned to Jersey. Some of his friends who were still in Jersey had written to him to say that the GPO (General Post Office) were taking men on because they had a large project in process they were laying underground cables. Bill got a job as a labourer and stayed there until Christmas when he came home to visit his family. Unfortunately, while he was at home his father collapsed and sadly died from a heart attack.

He rang the GPO in Jersey and told them what had happened. They sent wages owed to him plus his insurance cards; they also told him that if or when the time was right he could have his job back. Bill had to make all the arrangements because his mother wasn't coping very well. He had a younger brother who was still at school, and a younger sister who had not long started work. Because of his commitments at home, he couldn't go back to Jersey and he couldn't leave his mother.

So he applied for a job at the Unit Construction who had a large building project in the Halewood district of Liverpool and he was taken on as a labourer.

A couple of years after his father died, his mother hadn't been very well and spent some time in hospital, but it wasn't long before she came home and was able to look after her family once again. Sadly, a few short years later she collapsed and died. So once again, Bill had to make the necessary arrangements. Then he had to take care of his younger brother, and his sister had just become engaged. His other brother and sister were married with families of their own. Bill, like me, was the eldest in the family.

When he had finished telling me about himself, he looked at me, smiled, and said "That's where you come in Julia; it must have been fate" We both looked at each and laughed heartily together.

I was so surprised at what he said. It wasn't as if we were having a great love affair or anything like that, we'd only been out together half a dozen times. Nevertheless, we did get on with each other and enjoyed each other's company. We agreed he would come to the house and meet my family, the following Saturday.

Saturday evening Bill's car drew up outside my house. I went to the front door to greet him and invited him in. He followed me into the living room where Julianne and Catherine where sitting on the couch. Bill held his hand out to Catherine and said, "Hello love, how are you?" She took his hand, looked up at him and smiled, even though she couldn't speak her face lit up when he spoke to her. Julianne smiled at Bill and said hello.

Then my son Tony walked into the living room, he looked at me first, and then with a half smile said hello to Bill. Tony was nearly 18 by then.

I know it must have been difficult for him and I didn't expect him to understand. I would have liked to speak to him and explain but he wouldn't discuss anything with me.

Bill and I sat for a while and made awkward small talk. It seemed strange to me and it must have been the same for my family to see a man in the house. The only men who had been in my house since their father had died, were two of my brothers who would just call on me to see if we were alright.

With the initial greetings over with Bill and I decided to give it a go. Only time would tell if it would work out or not, but deep down inside my heart I knew it wasn't going to be easy.

~ 18 ~

"Three Times a Lady"

CHRISTINE'S HUSBAND Keith was a baker and worked at a small bakery in Garston. In the mean time he'd applied to a local major bakery in Speke and was offered a better job with more pay, which he gladly accepted. When he left, I took his place in the small bakery. Working in the tiny bakery was hard work but I enjoyed it because I use to bake a lot when the children were little. Of course, it was very different working in a bake house because there was far more baking to do. Once the baker had made the pastry my job was to roll it out on a pastry roller and then cut it with a special pastry cutter, which always reminded me of what my grandmother did on washing day.

She had a contraption which was called a mangle in the yard, which had two large wooden rollers and an enormous wrought iron handle. On washday, she'd place the wet sheets between the two large wooden rollers on the mangle. Then she'd take hold of the handle with two hands and turn it till the water ran out into a large galvanised bucket which stood underneath. After she'd folded and repeated the same motion the sheets would be ready to go onto the washing line!

Once I'd cut the pastry I'd place the prepared shaped pastry into their special tins and filled them with meat; same procedure applied with fruit pies, then I'd top them all, except for the custard tarts they didn't have to be topped.

I had to find a part time job because the widow's mother's allowance just wasn't enough. My hours were 6.30am until 12noon, I'd get home about twelve thirty and I'd just make myself a cup of tea, lay on the couch and fall asleep for most of the afternoon.

My son Tony had gone to Torquay for seasonal work; my brother Frank lived there at the time so I knew he'd be alright.

Christine had made a home of her own with her husband Keith and little son Antony. Julianne was sixteen years old, and Catherine was home at the weekends. I felt free and alive; I hadn't felt like that for such a long, long time.

About a year into our relationship, Bill moved in. We were going to see how things would work out between us because living with someone is far different from just seeing them twice a week.

One evening when Bill's sister and her husband were visiting us, she said unexpectedly "When are you two going to get married? I can see that you're just right for each other" Bill and I looked at each another and laughed.

Then Bill came right out with it and said, "What about it then babe shall we?"

I answered, "We might as well if it's only to stop the neighbours talking."

After shouts of joy and congratulations, we opened a bottle of "Martini Asti" that had been lying in the fridge since Christmas.

My daughter Christine was the first one I told about Bill and me getting married. She was overjoyed. She liked Bill and was glad that I had someone who cared about me the way he did. When I told Julianne she just smiled shrugged her shoulders and said it was fine by her. She was used to Bill because there was just the three of us in the house and Catherine at weekends. Julianne had a boyfriend and was out with him most of the time. I got in touch with my son Tony. He said he'd didn't mind but he wouldn't be at the wedding. I had to accept his wishes.

I told my parish priest that I was getting married in the registry office. He said that there was no need for me to get married in a registry office because it's cold and unfeeling. I said that I didn't think that I could get married in church again. He said that there was nothing to stop us getting married in church because I was a widow and Bill was a single man.

I told Bill when he came in from work and he was over the moon when I told him what the priest had said. He thought it was a great idea and said it would be much nicer to be married at the altar. Bill and I went to see the priest and he was delighted when we told him that we would like to marry in church. Both of us had to go to the priest's house for instructions a couple of times just to talk about my faith and to see if Bill had any objections to my faith, which he didn't. I was a Roman Catholic but not a practising one. Bill was a Baptist but not a practising one.

After all the arrangements were made I told my mum and dad that Bill and I had decided to get married and they were both very happy about it because they liked Bill.

A week or so later my father took me to one side and said, "Before you get married have you both talked about Catherine? Does Bill know what her needs are and always will be? Do you think he will be able to cope with it all? Have you both thought long and hard about it because it's not going to be easy? Are you absolutely sure?"

My exact words to him were "Yes of course I've told him all about Catherine. I introduced him to my family some time ago and he sees her when she's home at weekends and he was visibly upset when he saw her have a fit. I've been perfectly honest with him. But most importantly I've told him that Catherine and I will always be as one. As far as being sure about marrying Bill is concerned, I'm as sure as the sun will rise tomorrow, because he makes me feel very special dad. Above all there's no stress or anxiety and I feel safe and comfortable with him." Then I paused and said, "And you can give me away if you like."

He threw his head back, laughed and said, "OK Fair enough, if that's what you want."

Bill and I were married in St Christopher's Catholic Church at 3 0'clock on the 15th of August 1980. My dad gave me away and my two daughters Christine and Julianne were my maids of honour. They both looked beautiful in their new summer dresses and my little grandson Antony was my page. He looked so cute in his little page outfit. Catherine was on holiday at the time with Mencap. After the ceremony, we all stood on the steps of the church and had our photographs taken. We didn't have a professional photographer because both of our families had cameras. I had to take my high-heeled shoes off because I looked taller than Bill.

After the ceremony, we went straight into the church hall where a buffet was waiting and everything looked beautiful. My son Tony didn't come to the wedding; I did miss him and felt I wasn't complete without him. He'd told me that he wouldn't be coming but he did send us a telegram which read "All My Loving" I hadn't put him under any pressure because it had to be his decision. I still have the telegram. I knew that Bill and I would be seeing Tony the next day; because we were going to Torquay on our honeymoon and he was going to meet us from the train, so that made me feel a lot better.

Some old friends of Bill's came to our wedding, people he had known since teenage years; his sister had contacted them and he was delighted to see them.

I was especially happy that Christine, my late husband's sister, came to our wedding and joined in the celebrations. During the evening, she came over to where Bill and I were sitting and she wished us all the happiness and joy in the world. That meant a great deal to me because no matter what had happened between her brother and me, she and I had remained friends.

We had a disco for the evening's entertainment. The bar and hall was licensed until midnight so we had plenty of time to enjoy ourselves.

In a quiet moment, when everyone was on the dance floor or talking in his or her own little group, I reflected on the time when my late husband and I were married in the same church and at the same alter; and how we'd held our secret close to our hearts about me being pregnant.

It wasn't something you could talk about in 1958 so we had decided to get married with a promise to each other that we wouldn't mention it which was very hard. Both our parents badgered us about why we wanted to get married and what was the hurry, but we remained tight-lipped and never gave in.

November 8th 1958 was the day Tony and I were married. It was a cold but bright winter's day. There wasn't a buffet or anything like that but my mam and dad did their best and with the help of my grandmother, had made a lovely spread in my mother's living room. Covering the table was a snow-white sheet trimmed with lace with beautiful fresh flowers placed in the centre. At the top of the table was a gorgeous homemade wedding cake covered in white icing with tiny pink flowers in the middle. There was an egg and ham salad, a huge glass bowl filled with tinned fruit cocktail and a glass jug filled with cream. It really did look nice.

Discos didn't exist in 1958 so we all went to the local pub. Tony and I didn't care about those things then they didn't bother us. We loved one another very much and we just wanted to be together which was something both of our families didn't understand, but there again they didn't know that I was pregnant.

Tony's older brother Billy told us not to worry about having our wedding photographs taken because he had a good camera and he would be taking the photographs of our wedding, but he'd let us down when he didn't bring the camera. Having no photographs of our special day was a terrible disappointment and deep in my heart, I never forgave him for that because we had no photographs to show to our children.

We had to rely on friends and family to tell them why there were no photographs of our wedding. My mother and father were also very upset and angry because we had no photographic record of our marriage.

Our marriage had been a turbulent and stressful one; but the most precious gift that we'd achieved together was four beautiful children, and from those children five beautiful grandchildren, then three great grandchildren, so we must have done something right!

Bill woke me from my reverie as he sat down beside me and said "Penny for your thoughts Babe"

I cupped his face in my hands and said, "They're far more precious than that Bill, they're priceless." I grabbed his hand and said, "Listen to what they're playing. Come on, let's dance." It was the Commodores, *Three Times a Lady*. We joined the other couples on the dance floor. This was the song that Bill always sang to me, or tried to sing to me.

The next day my son-in-law Keith drove us to Lime Street station to catch the train for Torquay; we were going on our honeymoon.

I was looking forward to seeing my son and as we stepped from the train in Torquay, he was standing there on the platform. My heart leapt in my chest when I saw him. He looked so well and so very handsome. A big grin came over his face when he saw us.

Our train was running late and Tony had been back and forth to the station trying to find out what time it was expected. The porter had told him it was running at least three hours late and now that we'd arrived he had to hurry back to work but we'd made arrangements to meet later.

I know that it was hard for him to accept Bill. He wasn't a replacement father and never would be, that was out of the question. I just wanted Tony to accept Bill as a friend, not as a threat to my love for him. He was my son and I love him very much and always will. No man on this earth would never ever be able to take that love away from me no matter what happened. I prayed that maybe in time they'd become friends; well at least on speaking terms. I knew that it would take time and I understood that.

When we got back home after our honeymoon Bill went back to work; he was a forklift driver on a building site. I'd left my job at the bake house and was looking for something else.

One evening whilst Bill was reading the evening paper, there was an article about a little boy who'd had a road accident not as severe as Catherine's but bad enough. The article said that the little boy had been attending the BIBIC in Bridgewater, Somerset and over a matter of time had made remarkable progress. After talking about the article for some time Bill suggested I write to the BIBIC and ask if we could bring Catherine for an assessment. Well, they could only say yes or no!

The following morning I wrote my letter to the BIBIC explaining Catherine's injuries and how she'd received them, and how she was at the moment. About two anxious weeks later, we received our reply. Our appointment was for 9th September, 1981. This was just a couple of weeks after our first wedding anniversary. The next day I wrote back to the BIBIC and confirmed the time and date of our appointment; just like I did when my brother, mother, Catherine and I went to see the specialist at the Cambridge Hospital.

In the meantime, we noticed when Catherine came home for the weekend she always seemed to have a cold so instead of her enjoying her time with us we would spend the whole weekend getting her better. Throughout the following months, we talked about what we were going to do about the situation. We decided to finish with the residential care and bring her home. I wasn't working at the time so I would have more time to look after her.

Part Two

~ 19 ~

British Institute for Brain Injured Children

I WAS starting to feel very apprehensive as the day for our appointment drew near.

"What if its bad news again, Bill? What if there's nothing they can do to help her speak? I don't think I could I cope with another disappointment"

"Let's just wait and see. We'll cross that bridge when we get to it—nothing ventured nothing gained" he said in his laid back manner The journey there and back from Liverpool to Bridgewater in the same day was going to be a long one so we decided to have any early breakfast and leave for Somerset as soon as we were ready. Before we left we had to make sure that Catherine was tied securely and comfortable in the back seat, hoping that she wouldn't have a fit while we were travelling on the motorway. At last, we were ready. Our family and friends wished us well as we set out on our journey to the BIBIC in Somerset. I told my daughters Christine and Julianne about the wonderful work these people did and of course, they were supportive. I also wrote to my son Tony who lived and worked in London at the time.

After nearly four hours on the motorway, stopping to visit the toilet at a couple of service stations, we saw the signs for Bridgewater.

Then we took the slip road and looked for the sign that said Knowle Hall, where the BIBIC was. In the distance, we could see a large grey building, and on the side of the road, there was a sign pointing us in the right direction. Bill and I looked at one another and smiled. This was it. This was the place. We drove up the long gravel path to where a large impressive building stood surrounded by well-tended gardens. We were very impressed. The three of us got out of the car and were so relieved to be able to stretch our legs.

Catherine had some difficulty and moaned in pain. We rubbed her legs until her circulation improved and she was able to stand more steadily.

Bill and I held her hands and spoke to her, reassuring her that all was well. I don't think she liked the idea of going into this large building; it probably looked very intimidating to her.

As we opened the door of the Institute, we stepped into a beautiful hallway. The stone tiled floor pattern looked well worn where many feet had trodden over the years. There were a couple of doors on both sides of the hall and a broad staircase, which led to an upper floor. Through a large window halfway up the staircase, the autumn sun shone radiantly throwing its ray's over the splendour of the entrance hall. We sat on a bench that stood against the wall, a welcome rest for the weary and hopeful traveller.

No sooner had we sat down a door opened and a young woman walked toward us with a broad welcoming smile. She introduced herself as Mr. Pennock's secretary who was the director of the Institute and the man who we had come to see. She held out her hand to Catherine and said, "You must be Catherine. We've all been looking forward to meeting you! Would you and your parents like to come with me and meet Mr. Pennock?" Catherine smiled at her and stood up.

As we walked into his office, Mr. Pennock was standing behind his desk. He held his hands out and welcomed us to Knowle Hall. He was of slim build, and his hair was white and close cut with a neatly trimmed beard that complimented his well-tailored suit. After our brief introduction, Mr. Pennock said that he just wanted us to relax, have a cup of tea, and take it easy for a little while after our long journey from Liverpool. His secretary came into the room with a tray of freshly made tea and some biscuits.

As we sipped our tea, I was longing to take a biscuit and dunk it into my tea but I was scared stiff in case it fell into the cup—I would have died from embarrassment.

After we drank our tea, Mr. Pennock asked about Catherine's accident and apart from the obvious what were her injuries. We had spoken for some length when he asked; what was the most important question I would like to ask.

I told him that I needed to know why Catherine couldn't speak. Would she ever speak and was there anything that could give her a better quality of life because, I was very concerned about her future. I also told him what the doctor had said when her Father and I had taken her for her first assessment. He'd said that because of the accident and the injuries that she had sustained at that time, the full impact of those injuries had made clear that unfortunately she had suffered a stroke.

Mr. Pennock just looked at Catherine nodded his head and smiled. After we'd had our talk he suggested that we leave Catherine with him and certain members of his staff for a couple of hours so that they could assess her.

Bill and I agreed, after all that was the reason we were there. Before we left I spoke to Catherine and tried to explain to her what was happening and to reassure her that she was quiet safe and that Bill and I would be back very shortly. I didn't know if she understood but she smiled and waved to us as we left her in the care of the staff.

The drive to Bridgewater was only about fifteen minutes from Knowle Hall. After we'd parked the car we had a look around and thankfully found a tea-room. Over our hot buttered toasted teacakes and tea we talked about what the Institute might tell us on our return and hoped, and prayed that the news would be good.

After a couple of hours, we were weary of walking about Bridgewater and drove back to the Institute. As we pulled up outside we braced ourselves hoping for a good outcome from Catherine's assessment.

Mr. Pennock and his staff were waiting in his office for our return. Catherine didn't look upset or anything, and a big smile lit up her face as Bill and I walked into the room. Both of us sat on the edge of our seats waiting eagerly to see what Mr. Pennock was going to say.

Then he said, "In answer to your question about Catherine's inability to speak, I can tell you why she can't speak."

On hearing this, my heart nearly jumped out of my chest it was beating so fast. He continued, "Have you ever had a filling at the dentist? I replied that I had. "Ok then so the dentist puts a needle into your gum to deaden the tooth so that you don't feel anything?" Again, I said yes. "Well then, he continued, the reason why Catherine can't speak is because the inside of her mouth is partially paralysed; she can't taste or chew because she has no feeling on the inside of her mouth. And that is also the reason why she can't pull out her tongue because when she had her accident she'd also suffered a stroke"

I stared at him. I couldn't believe it sounded so simple. In such a short time he'd answered the questions that I'd been asking for the past eight years and everything he had said made sense. Then I remembered what the doctor told her father and me a few years ago when we'd taken her for an assessment after her accident. He had said that Catherine had had a stroke but had never explained to us why she couldn't speak, or if there was anything that could be done for her. Not one of the so-called experts had had a clue. My beautiful girl had been suffering all that time and couldn't tell us.

After hearing the news of Catherine's paralyses, Bill and I started firing questions at Mr. Pennock. Can he and his staff help? What could we do? When would we do it? How long would it take?

He sat on the edge of his desk looked at us both and said, "I and my staff can't make Catherine well again, but, we can work out a tailored programme just for her; in which we could try and teach her the skills that she had before the accident"

And so he began to explain what the programme would be. "This programme would consist of intense physical activities. First you will have to find 70 volunteers every week including yourselves. For the programme to be effective, you will have to work seven days a week. You will have to put yourselves and Catherine though a rigorous routine each day and every day. You will work as you've never worked before.

Bill and I looked at each other. I said "We'll do it; we'll try anything."

Bill nodded his head in agreement and said, "Whatever it takes we will do it."

Mr. Pennock shook his head and said, "No No No, I can't accept your answer so quickly. The first thing you must do is to talk it though with friends and family to find out if you can get the support that you need because believe me you are going to need it."

He finished by saying that there was also the financial cost, which was at that time, £128 every three months. Catherine had never received any compensation because at the time, I'd been given the wrong advice and it was too late. We left the BIBIC later that day with a bag of mixed feelings.

Before we began our journey back home, I called into a little shop that we'd passed on our way back from Bridgewater. I bought some snacks and drinks because they were very expensive at the motorway service stations.

I got Catherine out of the car and took her into the shop with me and Bill waited outside. It was a small grocery shop cum post office. I bought a box of Mr. Kipling country slices. Catherine could enjoy one or two of them if I broke them into tiny pieces. We always kept a clean tea towel, which I'd place onto her lap when I was giving her something to eat. I also kept plenty of tissues and a damp flannel in the glove compartment of the car. I bought some salt and vinegar crisps for Bill and me and a large bottle of lemonade. Catherine could manage a drink from a special baby cup that I'd bought for her.

As I passed my purchases to the woman at the till I turned and spoke to Catherine and said that we would be on our way home very soon. On hearing my accent, the woman looked at me and smiled and she asked me where I was from. "Liverpool" I said proudly.

I told her about the BIBIC and of course, she knew all about it. She said that she'd heard of people coming from all over the country and even from abroad to seek help and advice for their brain injured child. She said that Catherine was a beautiful young girl and that it would be just wonderful if there were a way to help her communicate.

I smiled and thanked her for her comments and just as we were about to walk out of the shop the woman said, "Please wait a minute."

She took a biro pen from the top pocket of her overall, wrote her name, address and phone number on a slip of paper, and handed it to me.

She said her name was Dot, and that she would be very pleased if or when we ever came back to the Institute, we would call on her and her husband as she would love to see Catherine again and would like hear about her progress. Just then, Bill came into the shop to see if we were alright. I introduced him to Dot and before we left I promised that the next time we were at the Institute I would ring her. I put the slip of paper in the side pocket of my shoulder bag and didn't think anymore about it, because my mind was full of what Mr. Pennock had told us.

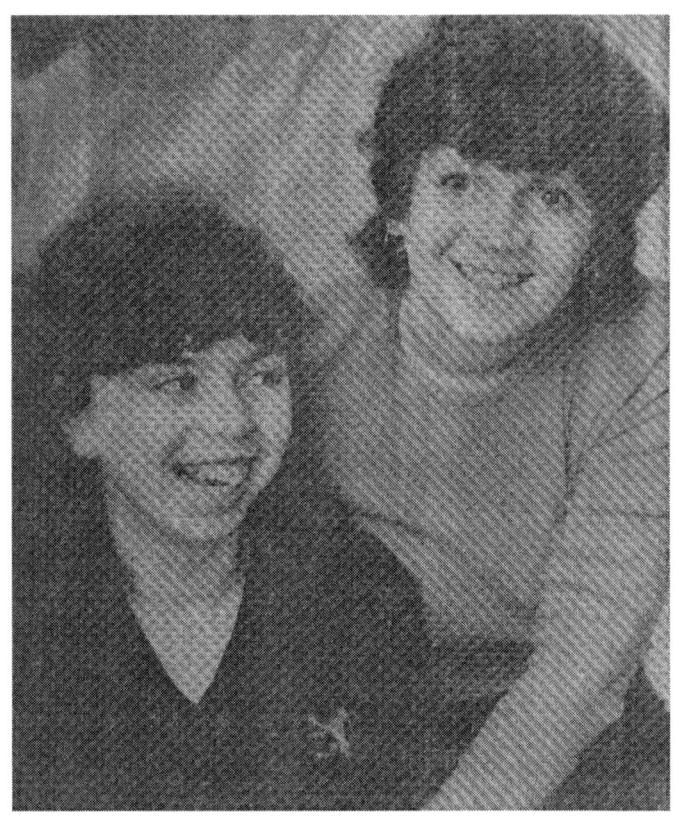

Catherine and her mother

~ 20 ~

Fundraising

A COUPLE of days after we'd arrived back home from the BIBIC we held a meeting with our family, friends and neighbours and all the people who had offered to help us. First thing that we had to do was raise some funds. Everyone was so supportive and said that they would do their best to help in any way that they could.

I went to see my local parish priest to ask if he had any idea, how I could acquire some volunteers and he said he would see what he could do. A few days later, I received a phone call from a man who said that he was working with The Liverpool Youth Service. He was helping some young people to work toward and achieve The Duke of Edinburgh Award. He said the priest had told him all about Catherine and what we we're trying to do. And he had spoken to a particular group of young people who were eager to come and help us. Then he said the volunteers who were going to come were taking part in the Duke of Edinburgh Award scheme. Also before they left I was to sign their form for them and explain how helpful they had been. I said that I most certainly would. So a group of four young people came to see us and there were more to follow.

One of my neighbours got in touch with two well-known local newspapers—the *Liverpool Echo* and the *Merseymart*. She told them all about Catherine and the Institute in Somerset. A few days later, both newspapers sent reporters out to interview us. We told them all about Catherine and with the help of our family, friends and neighbours, what we were trying to achieve.

They took some photographs of Catherine and me, and wrote about the help we needed and what we were trying to achieve for Catherine. Just a week later, the story and photographs appeared in both papers.

The solicitor to whom I had gone to seek advice from, regarding of what to do and how to keep accounts if and when people sent us money for our cause, joined us in our campaign and a couple of weeks later did a sponsored parachute jump for us.

A couple of girls who worked at the Maypark Chicken Factory

came to see us and offered to do a charity night, which to our delight they did.

Then a couple of young men rang and said they were going to do a sponsored swim. St Christopher's social club, which adjoined to St Christopher's school in Stapleton Avenue and the school that Catherine had attended before the accident arranged a charity night.

Some local residents had adopted the Merseymart Running Team to raise money for "The Catherine Kehoe Fund" in the London Marathon, which was going to take place on 21st April.

All these offers of help gave Bill and me the encouragement to carry on. There were so many people whose names I couldn't possibly recall after all these years but whose kindness was overwhelming. If any of those supporters involved with us at that time are reading this book, I am sure that they will remember.

We sent all the cheques and money to the Institute and each, and every one, received a receipt. If any anonymous money arrived I would make a date of it in my accounts and send it off to Somerset, who would then send me a receipt and I would entre it in my ledger. Nearly four months later, from the time we had began our campaign, we our family and friends had raised enough money to begin our therapy.

Those volunteers who were going to start the first week of the programme with Bill and I came to see us and decided the day and date that they could come. Once we had received commitments from our family, friends and neighbours, Bill made a rota of the volunteer names, with what day and time they were coming and placed on the living room wall.

In due course, I wrote to Mr. Pennock at the Institute and told him that with the help of our family, friends and neighbours, we had raised enough money and had everything organised to the best of our ability and felt that we were ready to begin Catherine's programme.

About a week later, we received a letter congratulating us all for organizing so much in so short a time. They also gave us a date when we were to visit the Institute to learn the programme for Catherine's treatment. They said we would have to stay for a full week because it would take that amount of time for us to learn and take in all that we had to do in the first four months. Two afternoons during that week we would be attending lectures about brain injury and what if anything can be done, depending of course on the severity of the injury.

They also sent us an address for a bed and breakfast, which was very close by. We couldn't stay at the Institute for our learning week, but when we returned for our four monthly assessments we would be able to stay overnight. I wrote to the B and B and arranged our weeks stay.

After an early breakfast on the following Sunday morning we began our journey to Somerset because the next morning at nine sharp we would have to be at the Institute to begin Catherine's programme.

When we arrived at Knowle we found the address were we were to stay for the week. The lady of the house made us very welcome. She used to work at the Institute so she knew what our hopes and dreams were.

After breakfast and a very, sleepless night, the three of us set off on our five-minute journey. On our arrival, we went into what looked like a gym. There were also three other sets of parents with their brain injured child. We smiled nervously at one another and made small talk while we waited in anticipation for Mr. Pennock and his staff to arrive. Then at nine o'clock, the staff walked in all bright and breezy and greeted us all with a warm welcome. We looked at each other not knowing what to expect. We were about to find out.

Learning How to Do the Patterning

THE PROGRAMME we were about to learn, was based on The Doman Delacto Therapy whose main base was in Philadelphia in the USA. In principal, the therapy patterns the brain into learning skills; skills that Catherine already had before the accident and with patterning would hopefully return.

Some children were more disabled than others were but nevertheless that didn't make any difference, we all were treated equally. We were about to start the most arduous week of our lives.

The first exercise was to get Catherine onto what they called a patterning table. To do this patterning five people had to take part; one was to hold her head gently, two for her arms and two for her legs. As she lay face down on the patterning table, the five volunteers in unison would move her head arms and legs into a walking position; it was so very difficult at the start. With three staff members, Bill, me, and Catherine protesting very loudly, we eventually got into the rhythm. While we patterned Catherine, we recited nursery rhymes together. Miss Polly Had a Dolly was one of her favourites. This patterning would last just five minutes.

Looking back it must have felt more like an hour to Catherine. The patterning would start each session and there were four sessions every day. The correct descriptions for the volunteers was, "Patteners"

There were many more important physical activities to be done after the patterning table session. The next activity was the crawl box, which we hoped would teach her to crawl again. Crawling was a skill that she already knew before the accident but even though she began to walk again a year after the accident, she walked very badly and with a notable gait. However, Catherine had missed the crawling stage of development so we hoped it would pattern her brain with this experience.

Then there was the spatial awareness exercise. This was where we placed Catherine in a large wicker basket chair, which hung from a bracket from the centre of the monkey ladder. Then under protest from Catherine, we slowly swung her around one way then another.

Then Bill had to pick Catherine up by her waist with his two hands and hold her under the monkey ladder. I must add that at that time she was very slim and only four foot nine. Then one of the staff and I placed her hands on the rungs of the ladder and tried to encourage her to grasp the rungs just as children do when they play on the monkey ladder in the park. This was another spatial awareness exercise. In between all these activities, we would have to show her some flash cards, which we were to make ourselves.

Then there were the tactile exercise where I had to stroke some small pieces of rough and smooth, then hot and cold material gently onto her hands, face and under her feet.

Then we teased her taste buds, because she didn't have much feeling inside her mouth. I had to place something sweet then something sour onto her tongue, any two different tastes six times a day. The optimism was this would enable Catherine to once again taste her food and stop the dribbling and maybe, just maybe, please God, enable her to speak, no matter how poorly.

Next, a member of the staff showed us how to place a small see through plastic mask over Catherine's nose and mouth just for a few seconds.

This was to see if it would improve her breathing. This like the other procedures, repeated six times a day. I must point out that Bill and I were in constant attendance at all times.

The principal of the therapy was to start all over again, from lying on the floor—to crawl—to stand—and then to walk.

Two afternoons throughout that particular week, Mr. Pennock spoke to us all about what happens when a brain injury occurs. This discussion was very informative, also, a very welcome break from the patterning table. First, he explained that our brains are a beautiful pink coral colour; and little grey cells only occur when we are dead. The brain is a magnificent organ and dictates every move we make, and it controls all of our emotions.

After following a multi-disciplinary assessment week, we were ready to return home. Before we left, we had to see Mr. Pennock. He said that at first when we begin the programme at home, we might find it harder to do because the staff wouldn't be there to help.

Moreover, he continued that in such a short time, just a week, we had done very well and he was confident that we would do everything to the best of our ability. And, to always remember that he and the staff were only on the other end of the phone. He said that we'd be sent an appointment at the end of three months to bring Catherine back for an assessment to see if there had been any improvement in her condition. Before we left, he added that we had to follow the programme to the letter and not leave anything out.

Once parents and their volunteers began the therapy at home, their progress would be carefully monitored. A member of staff from the BIBIC would call to see the families at home just to make sure that all is well, and programmes would be adjusted as and when necessary.

After our parting talk with Mr. Pennock, he and the staff waved us good-bye and wished a safe journey back home to Liverpool. Armed with Catherine's programme and all that we had learn a surge of excitement ran though me. I was eager to start. As soon as we arrived home, we were going to call a meeting with our family, friends and neighbours.

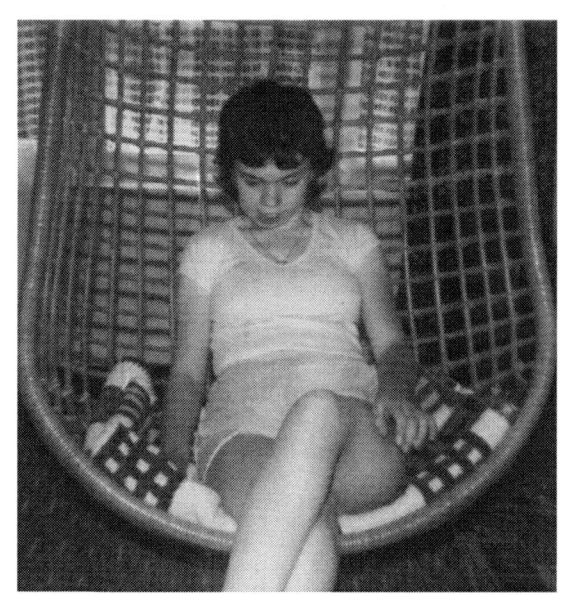

Beginning the Doman Delacto Therapy
Programme

~ 22 ~

Making the Adaptations

WHEN BILL and I got married, we brought Catherine home for good instead of just weekends. She had been in residential care Monday-Friday for about fourteen months. Bill and I were going to put all our energies into trying to get Catherine better.

Just before our visit to Somerset, Bill lost his job through redundancy. Strange as it might seem everything seem to fall into place because I couldn't have possibly done it all on my own. We needed to work closely together and we both had to show the volunteers' what to do.

The day before we were going to start the programme Bill and I ran though our schedule. We went over and over it repeatedly. We had to be sure we knew what we were doing. It was essential to keep to the programme tailored especially for Catherine as planned. We had to work out how long each of the session would take because we had four to complete each day.

First, there was the patterning table – five minutes.

Small see through mask – one minute.

Crawl box – five to six minutes.

Then, while Catherine was having a break and while she was sitting in the chair, I did my tactile with some soft and slightly rougher material on her face, then the front and back of her hands and under her feet using two different materials every day.

Then we would have a coffee break. Catherine could have a cup of tea or juice – fifteen minutes

Then the monkey ladder – five minutes.

Then Bill would fix the wicker chair to the bracket on the monkey ladder and place her in the wicker chair – five minutes.

Then after given lots of praise and shouts of joy for Catherine at the end of each session, which I must add was part of the programme, we would have a fifteen coffee break and toilet.

There had to be four sessions each day, two mornings and two afternoons. All in all, each session could take ten to fifteen minutes longer depending on Catherine's co-operation.

We knew that the first week would be hit, and miss, until we got into the rhythm of the programme. We would have to show each volunteer what to do, and sometimes if one of our regulars couldn't make it we have to show the person who had come in their place; which could be time consuming but nevertheless we had to have our volunteers. Once they and we were confident, we could carry on without having to explain everything two or three times a day

After running through the written programme for an hour or so, Bill and I placed each piece of equipment at the top end of the living room. We placed the patterning table, which was 6ft long and 3ft wide and usually stood in the middle of the room, (Catherine is 4ft 9inches) against the wall for the time being because it was in the way and brought it back out for each patterning session.

The patterning table was given to us by a family who lived in Litherland, who had finished the therapy and whose daughter had done very well. They also gave us a metronome and a breathing harness ready for when we got to a further stage in the programme. They said that doing the therapy could be very harrowing at times, but nevertheless they encouraged us to give it a try.

Bill's best friend Jack was a fantastic help and was always so supportive in our quest to get Catherine well again. Jack worked in the engineering department at The Metal Box Factory in Speke. He had spoken to his boss at the factory where he worked and explained what we were trying to achieve and what equipment we needed, like the crawl box, the ladder for the ceiling, and all the brackets needed to secure them to the living room wall and ceiling. His boss listened with interest and said that he would see what he could do. A couple of days later Jacky's boss came to see him and asked him what were the measurements of the equipment that we needed, because he'd got permission to make them.

Jack called in to see us on his way home from work and told us his good news. His boss was willing to help us. He also said they would supply some of the stiff card that we needed to make our flash cards. Once again, Bill and I were amazed at the kindness and generosity shown to us.

I appealed on our local radio station to the Billy Butler Show on Radio Merseyside; just to see if there was anyone who happened to have a large hanging wicker chair that swung from the ceiling which they didn't need any more. The next day I received four offers; even a businessman who was driving on the motorway at the time, rang the radio station and offered to buy us one. Once again, we were overwhelmed by how so many people, people who didn't even know us, wanted to help. We decided to accept the one that was kindly offered by a lady in Childwall, which was only fifteen minutes by car from where we lived.

A couple of days before we began the therapy, Bill and his friend Jacky had fitted the monkey ladder securely across the living room ceiling. Then they placed a bracket in the middle of the ladder to hang the large wicker chair when needed; which would be four times a day. Then when the therapy is finished for the day, the chair could be unhooked and placed on top of the patterning table at the end of the living room. The bracket was also used for the part of the programme when we'd wrap a thick strap around Catherine's ankles and suspended her upside down. While she was in that position I would lay underneath her and the volunteers would sit on the floor around her. As this was happening we'd play disco music and we'd all try to encourage her to swing, this was part of her spatial awareness. I know that this sounds so cruel but this and the wicker chair would hopefully help her with her spatial awareness.

Then there was the crawl box, which was eight foot long, two foot wide and eighteen inches high. Along the top of the crawl box on each side, two-inch holes were drilled and through the holes we placed broom handles, there were about twelve in all. The purpose of the crawl box was to keep Catherine on her tummy on the floor so that she would have to crawl out, which at that time was something she couldn't do.

Even though she had began to walk she had missed out the skill of crawling because she couldn't do it due to her brain injury, so hopefully we could pattern her brain and show her how to do it again.

I was to crawl though the box first; then Bill and the volunteers would try to encourage Catherine to follow me through the crawl box by clapping and cheering until hopefully she would do it herself. No matter if she couldn't do what we were trying to get her do on the programme, we praised her for everything that she did do, no matter how big or small.

The law of nature determines that in our first year of life we must follow the pattern set for us. From the floor, we crawl, from crawling we stand and then we walk.

I know that what we were doing for Catherine sounds cruel, but believe me it wasn't. What I do know that at first it was very difficult for her because she didn't quite understand what we were doing; but our smiles, kiss's and shouts of praise made it all a lot better and I knew she understood that.

~ 23 ~

Dedication and Commitment

THE DAY we were to start Catherine's programme arrived. Bill was out of bed first at 6:30am. He woke me with a smile and a cup of coffee and said, "Come on love, today's the day. We'll have to have an early breakfast because we have to get the equipment ready and there's lot to do before the volunteers arrive."

With my eyes still closed and my legs hanging over the edge of my bed, I sipped my coffee slowly. Images of what we were about to do, brought me to my senses and I was suddenly wide-awake.

When I went into Catherine's room, she was awake and lifted her hand out to me. I told her that it was time to get up and have our breakfast because we were going to have a very busy day.

After we'd had our showers and eaten, Bill and I began to put our equipment in place. Just to make sure that Catherine would be comfortable while doing her first day's therapy, I dressed her in shorts and t-shirt. When all was ready, Bill placed the rota on the living room wall. Our first volunteers would hopefully be the three young people who had come to see us a couple of weeks ago, the ones who were doing the Duke of Edinburgh Award, and told us what days they would be available.

While we waited for our volunteers to arrive, Bill and I spoke to Catherine and did our best to explain what we were about to do and why we were doing it. Just then and to our relief our three young volunteers arrived on time 9 o'clock. We could never have started the programming without them.

So we began our quest to improve Catherine's quality of life. When she co-operated the day would be just wonderful and at those times, we always felt that she had taken a step forward. Sometimes, and understandably so, she could be very difficult and we'd have to try and encourage her to carry on. That worked most time but sometimes it just didn't.

Bill and I did understood how she must have felt. Doing those same physical exercises day in and day out must have been very tiring for

Catherine, but we had to continue. We were committed to Catherine gaining as much independence as possible, but she didn't understand. How could she?

24

We Begin to See Results

THE FIRST four months of doing the therapy had been very taxing for us all, but then, and just before we were to go for our first assessment at the BIBIC, Catherine made a significant improvement—she had learned to crawl on her stomach!

Mr. Pennock and all the staff at the Institute were absolutely, delighted when she did it for them at her assessment on 8th June 1982. They clapped, cheered and congratulated her—and us as too. They also said, to our delight, that we didn't have to use the crawl box anymore and we didn't have to use the small plastic mask anymore. Instead, we were to use the breathing harness with the metronome for timing. This new exercise had to be five times a day, one with each of her four sessions and then half an hour in the evening. The evening procedure done as Catherine lay on her back on the patterning table.

Before we left, they gave us a new task to do, which was to help Catherine to crawl on her hands and knees on her own without falling over. That's where Bill's homemade harness came in! We decided it was also time to make our own flash cards.

Mr. Pennock suggested that we buy large posters, which had pictures of different objects such as, cats, dogs, birds, insects, articles of clothing, toys etc; anything that was bright and informative. The card had to measure 12 inches by 12 inches.

Before we left the institute, they presented Catherine with an achievement award for learning how to crawl on her stomach in her first four months on the therapy. Then two weeks later, just as we were about start of our second four monthly assessments we received a letter to say that Catherine's name was now entered into the book of achievements and on display in the front hall of the Institute. Both our volunteers and we were elated; it gave us all the incentive to continue with the programme.

I must say that at the beginning of each day I'd find myself getting very anxious just in case any of our volunteers were a bit late. Maybe their bus was late, or something had happened at home and they couldn't come, but if they knew before hand they would always ring. I have to say, they'd do their best to get someone to cover for them because they knew that we wouldn't be able to do the exercises without the three volunteers in attendance.

Of course, Bill and I were always there. Catherine's two sisters Christine and Julianne were also on the rota and would always stand in for us if someone couldn't come.

My grandson Antony would sometimes come with his mother Christine when he was on school holidays, and as young as he was he would help as well. My mother and father were also on the rota and if a volunteer couldn't come my parents would come and stand in for them. They only lived around the corner from where we lived so that was just fine.

My son Tony had gone to live in London. Nevertheless, I always let him know how Catherine was doing and I'd send him a copy of her assessment from the BIBIC.

I must also mention my lovely next-door neighbours Mr. and Mrs. Burns, who had put up with all the noise while we were doing the therapy. She told me not to worry about any noise; we were to just carry on and try to do our best for Catherine.

Our Second Fourth Monthly Session

NOW THAT the crawl box was thankfully finished with, Bill made a pair of shorts from an old pair of Catherine's jeans. One of my neighbours, a wiz on the sewing machine, sewed two straps on the back of the shorts, which was fantastic. This meant that Bill and I could grab a strap each and walk up and down the living room with Catherine inside the harness, until hopefully and eventually she would be able to crawl on her hands and knees without support. We did these four times a day, once with each session.

Then there was the breathing harness, with timing from the metronome. After her shower in the evening, Bill and I would place Catherine on her back onto the patterning table, but before we did this, we'd tie a special harness around her chest which had two straps one either side. Once this was done Bill and I would stand facing each other across the table; then we'd turn the metronome on and gently pull on the harness in time with a nice gentle heart beat. It was very important to keep time because we were trying to help her breath deeper, which hopefully would curb the dribbling and contribute to her speaking. Bill and I did this procedure every evening at 7 o'clock. Having said that, my neighbour Carol and her husband Jimmy who lived opposite us, who were also volunteers, would come over two evenings a week to give us a break on the harness.

Every evening after the breathing harness section was finished Bill and I would cut some pictures out of the posters and make our flash cards of different categories. Over a matter of weeks, we had accumulated quite a lot, and I might add, very well made for the amateurs we were. So in between the patterning table, then tactile, face, hands and feet, then wicker chair and monkey ladder, I'd show her the flash cards six times a day.

And so we carried on, day by day, working toward Catherine's next assessment.

I noticed that she seemed to enjoy looking at the flash cards. I would look at her eyes every time I showed her the card and had a feeling she was beginning to recognise some of the pictures I'd shown her.

Moreover, something else I noticed, because of the tactile sessions I was doing with her face her lovely smile seemed to be getting a little straighter. I prayed silently to myself that slowly but surely, my little girl was on her way to being a bit more independent.

Over the following weeks, Catherine, with the help of the harness, was crawling much quicker, so much so Bill could hold the harness without me because she wasn't putting her whole weight onto it. And so, with lots of claps and plenty of praise her confidence grew, then if she got too excited she would just slip and fall to the side, then we'd all laugh and thankfully so would she. Then before we knew it, we received our appointment for Catherine's next assessment. Sometimes our appointment would be for a Monday morning; which was really, good for us because we could travel down Sunday and stay overnight at the Institute.

When we arrived at the Institute in Somerset, and out of the blue, my son Tony had come to meet us. He had driven up from London and we overjoyed to see him. I had written to him previously to let him know how Catherine was progressing. When it was our turn to go in for Catherine's assessment, and before he left, I told Tony that I would let him know the result of Catherine's assessment and with a fond goodbye, he drove away.

WE WAITED in the gym for the staff to come and assess Catherine.

After showing them, all she had achieved since our last visit the staff were very pleased with her. Then, when a member of staff showed Catherine the flash cards, she picked out each one correctly. These were the cards and pictures that I'd been showing to her every day. Mr. Pennock and his staff also congratulated Bill on his specially made harness, they said it was the best they had ever seen, and he should patent it. Bill just laughed. So that was a feather in Bills cap and rightly so because he had worked so hard. By the end of this assessment, he had other things to make which I must say to his credit, he did and with great care and precision.

When the assessment was finished we were given other tasks to do mostly to do which were mainly exercises for Catherine's mouth, like blowing, sucking and lip movements, which were to be done in front of a mirror.

Even though Catherine had made great strides by crawling on her hands and knees, she still couldn't do it without the harness, so we were to carry on with that, also the flash cards, tactile, wicker chair and monkey ladder.

When we got back home, we called our volunteers together and told them what we were to do next; and so a few days later we began again.

25

The Nuffield Hospital, Oxford

AFTER ABOUT a year on the programme; Bill and I spoke to Mr. Pennock's secretary at the Institute and asked was there anything that could done to help Catherine walk a bit better and maybe improve her balance.

She said that she would write to The Nuffield Hospital in Oxford and request an appointment with an orthopaedic specialist. She said that she would also explain about the therapy that we were administering to Catherine, and hopefully, rather than making a separate journey, she asked if there were possibility that the appointment could coincide at the same time as our assessment at the Institute. To our delight, the hospital understood the practicalities of our travelling. The appointment they gave us meant that after our assessment at the Institute we could travel on from Somerset to Oxford. Dr Pennock's secretary also gave us the address of The Red Mullions Hotel where we could stay overnight, and which was close to our appointment at Nuffield hospital.

When we arrived at the Hotel, the staff gave us a very warm welcome. As we chatted, we told them why we were keeping this hospital appointment with the orthopaedic specialist and all about Catherine and the Institute in Somerset. As we left for the hospital, the following morning the staff at the hotel wished us well and hoped that they would see us again because we were going to go straight home to Liverpool after our appointment.

When we arrived at Nuffield, I gave Catherine's name to the receptionist, then a nurse showed us into a cubicle were we were to wait for the doctor. After a long wait and trying to reassure Catherine, that everything would be alright. She didn't like being behind the curtains because she couldn't see what was going on. Then at last the cubical curtains swished back and the specialist came in accompanied by his two assistants.

After the general chitchat, we explained about Catherine's accident and the therapy that we were doing. Then he said, "Ok then Catherine,

I would just like to have a look at your legs and see if there is anything we can do for you."

Then he asked Bill and me to lift her up onto the bed. She protested loudly as we both struggled to lift her up onto the narrow bed. Eventually, after we'd calmed her down, the doctor examined her legs, or I should say he tried to, because she didn't like the pressure of his hands but the doctor was patient with her and carried on with his examination.

After he'd finished his examination he said that he was going to make a splint for Catherine's left leg, but also, which wasn't going to be easy, she would have to keep it on when she went to bed because over time it may just straighten her leg, but he couldn't promise that it would.

So she was measured for the splint, again, under protest. He said once the splint was ready an appointment would be sent because she would have to try the splint on to make sure it was a comfortable fit. So at least we had some sort of a result but we would just have to see how and if she copes with it.

About six weeks later, we received at letter from the Nuffield hospital to say that Catherine's splint was ready. I rang The Red Mullions Hotel and reserved a room for the night before our appointment. We'd been given a late afternoon slot and didn't fancy driving there and back to Oxford on the same day. It would give us some time to have a look around Oxford.

We sat in anticipation in the waiting room eager to see what the splint would be like. After a little while, they called Catherine's name. We followed the nurse into the cubicle where the doctor and his students were waiting for us.

He greeted us with a smile and said "Hello Catherine, how are you? Would you like to try this splint on for me? It's been made especially for you. She looked at the splint then she looked at me and even though she couldn't speak her eyes were saying NO CHANCE! Amid protest and coaxing words from Bill and me, we managed to place her foot on the slim platform and ease the back of the splint onto the back of Catherine's leg, just up to her calf. Then we wrapped a broad elastic bandage around her foot and up her leg. She didn't like it at all, but we all understood. She had never worn anything like it before and it must have felt so strange.

After promising that we would do our best to get Catherine to wear the splint in bed, we left the hospital with mixed feelings. We both knew that it was going to be very difficult but we'd have to try; maybe she would get used to it and maybe she wouldn't. We made our way back to the hotel to pick up our bags and say our good-byes.

The owner of the hotel and a couple of the staff came out and wished us a safe journey home, and just as we were about to leave, the owners young daughter gave Catherine a mixed bag of chocolate treats for the journey. As we drove away from the hotel, I took the treats from her and put them away in the glove compartment. I couldn't leave them with her because she may have tried to eat them while we were driving and choke.

Every night was trial and error with the splint. As Bill and I fitted the splint onto her leg each night, we'd try and explain to her why we were doing it. Sometime's after I'd put her to bed at night I would hear a slight thud on her bedroom floor and would go upstairs to see what was happening. The splint would be lying on the floor or on the chair at the side of her bed and she would just look up and smile at me. For the next few weeks, we did our best to persevere but she was a determined young woman and wasn't going to give in without a fight. After two or three very trying months, we had to give in.

I wrote to the Nuffield Hospital and explained the situation, how it was beginning to become stressful for the three of us. The orthopaedic doctor wrote back and said that he understood how difficult it must have but at least we tried. So that was the end of the splint, nothing ventured nothing gained.

THROUGHOUT THE following year and during our assessments at the BIBIC they gave us many mouth exercises to do which were.

1. A mouth organ to encourage blowing:

2. Another blowing exercise:

Bill bought small plastic 10 centre meters tubing and cut it into three pieces so that we each had a piece and then fill a large bowl with water. Then he and I would blow into the water, make bubbles, and try to encourage Catherine to join in.

3. Then there were the mouth exercises. We would pull faces in front of a mirror and by pursing our lips and make whoooooo—eeeeeeeee sounds, and then grimace, and then we'd clap our hands and laugh and try to make it fun.

4. Then there was the book of speech rhymes which we

bought from BIBIC. We used to try to make it fun reciting the speech rhymes and pulling faces because some of them were humorous and over time, she began to make some meaningful sounds.

Then there were the hand and eye co-ordination exercises.

1. Bill took a length of wood, eighteen inches in length and six inches in width. Then he made a graph from a wire hanger and a small loop that Catherine was to hold and move along the wire without touching it.

2. Next, he cut out the bottom and most of the surround of a plastic bucket, which just left about a third of the bucket. Then he attached and pinned an onion net to the rim. Then he tacked it onto18inch wooden board and placed it onto the living room wall; and there we had it, our own hand made basketball net.

3. Next piece of equipment that Bill made was a dartboard. He made this by using a lid of a plastic tub, which he divided into four quarters and covered them with different coloured materials and he placed it onto the living room wall. Next, he bought half dozen table tennis balls and put strips of Velcro around them; which meant, that when Catherine threw a ball at the board it would stick, well done to my creative husband.

Although the last eighteen months had been very taxing, Catherine had made a most significant improvement, which was the return of her taste buds. This was the result of the different tastes I'd been putting onto her tongue six times a day; like salt, vinegar, bitters, anything that had a strong taste. I'll never forget the day that it happened. I'd squirted some lemon juice into her mouth, and then to our amazement, she screwed up her face from the bitter taste of the lemon juice. We all jumped about clapped and cheered and told her how wonderful and clever she was. This was fantastic and we felt so victorious. Her future looked brighter; it was such a wonderful achievement and she'd be able to enjoy the taste her food again!

I rang the Institute and told Mr. Pennock what had happened and he was as excited as we were. He said we were to praise her and tell her how wonderful she is. I laughed and said yes, we already have. I cried for joy and I thanked God from the bottom of my heart; to Bill and I this was a miracle. Having regained her taste buds and over the coming months Catherine started to take some control over her dribbling.

When the appointment came for Catherine's assessment we excited and so looking forward to seeing Mr. Pennock and the staff. We were eager to show them what our daughter had achieved. Of course, the team were full of praise for her. Mr. Pennock said how hard we must have worked to get such a very important result in such a short time. He said he was going to put Catherine's name in the book of achievements, which stood on a table in the entrance hall for all to see.

During her assessment, she had a word recognition test. Well, we just couldn't believe it when she read some single words. I always felt that she could recognise some words because when I'd shown her the flash cards during her therapy sessions she seemed to recognise them but I wasn't too sure.

Before we left the staff congratulated Bill and I and applauded our selfless volunteers. This wonderful progress gave us the encouragement to carry on. I couldn't express how proud and happy Bill and I felt.

On our return home, we told everyone how Catherine's assessment went and about her award. They were ecstatic because every one of our volunteers had a hand in Catherine's continuous progress.

Over the next four months, we were to carry on with the same routine; there was no change in her programme this time around. We were to wait till the next appointment which would be in four months time and then probably if all went we would move on to the next stage. With the exception of putting, different tastes on her tongue, and to keep on trying to encourage her to drink thorough a straw. We were all so pleased that Catherine's assessment was positive.

~ 26 ~

Bringing Home the Scrumpy

BEFORE WE left Somerset, we decided to find the farm, which we'd noticed during our travels back and forth to Bridgewater. We wanted to buy some Scrumpy for some of our young volunteers because we'd promised them that we would and before we left they said that it had to be "the good stuff!" After driving around for a little while, we eventually found the farm. A man who I presumed was the farmer came out of the barn when he heard us drive in. I couldn't help but notice that there was an awful sweet and sour smell about the yard which made me feel a little nausea.

When Bill told him, what we wanted and whom it was for, the farmer gave a loud and hearty laugh. "Oh yeah" he said, "I've got the right one for you. I'll mix some medium with a little strong, which will give it a good kick!" Then he asked Bill to follow him. I stood by the car with Catherine, looked around the yard, and thought what an awful mess! Even though the mounds of apples, which were beginning to go brown, were all stacked neatly, it nearly put me off my love of my apples for good, which was and always will be English Cox Pippin.

A few minutes later Bill and the farmer came out of the barn. The farmer was holding a one-gallon plastic container; I presumed filled with the Scrumpy. As he handed the container to Bill he said that before we set off for home he was to make sure that the container was secured good and proper and wasn't able to roll about in the boot. It was important that we stopped now and again to unscrew the cap to let the air out because it could explode. When the farmer saw the look of horror on my face, he burst out laughing and said, "Now don't you worry my dear, everything will be just fine. Your husband has it all in hand,"

So, to be on the safe side and to prevent me from having a heart attack Bill smiled at me and said, "Come on it'll be alright. I'm going to take the A roads so that I can stop and check it. Then after shaking hands with the farmer we drove away. As promised, Bill took the A roads and kept stopping to check the container. Throughout the entire journey home, I kept waiting for the big bang, which thankfully never came!

A few days later when our young volunteers arrived for duty, we told them that we had bought the Scrumpy they'd wanted. To say they were happy would be an understatement!

The following week when the same young men whom we had bought the Scrumpy for said that they and a couple of their friends had gone to Sefton Park and shared the potent brew. They said that after drinking it all between them they had fallen asleep on the grass and had lain there until dusk. Nevertheless, they said it was great fun and a great buzz.

On hearing this, I was horrified. Something terrible could have happened. Therefore, I told them that I wasn't going to buy them anymore. Needless to say, they were very disappointed, but I just wasn't going to take the chance after realising something terrible could have happened to one of them.

So that was the end of the Scrumpy!

27

Catherine Joins a Swimming Club

OVER THE next couple of years Catherine's programme changed; some things taken out and new ones added. The main thing was, and I must say to our great relief, the patterning table was taken off the programme, also the evening breathing harness because she was beginning to have more control over her dribbling. When the patterning table went in a way, it was a blessing. Some of our volunteers came and went; some were students who understandably had to carry on with their studies and some had changed their jobs and worked different hours so sometimes they just couldn't come. With the patterning table gone, we just needed two volunteers to work with Bill and me. If we were short of hands, Catherine's two sisters, Christine and Julianne, who were already on the rota, were always there to give us their support when we needed it. My mother and father also still helped us out and were still on the weekly rota.

In the mean time, we had joined an evening swimming club that was just for young people with learning difficulties. It was just wonderful because there weren't any members of the public jumping in and screaming, which would frighten Catherine and her friends. I always got into the water with her and encouraged her to follow me, which in time she did.

One evening and without warning, she swam away from me. I panicked because we were in the deep end, which was ten foot deep. She swam into the centre. I tried to keep calm as I swam toward her because I wasn't a very good swimmer and I pulled her back toward the bar. When we reached the bar, everybody clapped and told her how brave she was and she just smiled. She had her armbands on at all times because she couldn't swim without them.

A couple of weeks later the person who ran the club presented Catherine with an endeavour award. The class was only for one hour a week, but one hour well spent, because not only was it good exercises for her legs it was building up her confidence in the water.

At our next assessment at the Institute, we told the staff that

Catherine had joined a swimming club but also stressed that I was always with her in the water and that she always wore her armbands. And how as the weeks went on she had became more confidant in the water, so much so that one evening she swam away from me and had received a plaque for endeavour from the swimming club manager.

The team were delighted to hear our news and presented Catherine with another achievement award.

AT THE beginning of the third year on the programme, we gave Catherine three new exercises to do to which we hoped would improve her balance

The three new exercises were:

1. To encourage her to hold a pen and get her to write by following dot-to-dot letters;

2. To help her to walk a balance beam:

3. Was to be stepping-stones:

So once again, we turned to Bills friend Jacky who worked at The Metal Box Company in Speke. They had already made us some of the specialised equipment that we needed when we first began the programme.

When we explained to Jacky what we needed. He said he would approach his boss and ask if they would be able to help us again. Thankfully, his boss agreed to help, within a couple of weeks Jacky delivered the equipment we needed.

The balance beam was seven foot long and eight inches wide. With Bill on one side and me on the other, we would hold Catherine's hands while she walked the beam, then turn and walk back, six times a day.

Then treading the stepping-stones, consisting of five large one-foot square, wooden boxes, again, Bill and I held her hands as she stepped from box to box, also done six times a day. The same principal applied to both the balance beam and stepping-stones until she could do these tasks unaided, which in time she did.

And so, we carried on with the programme which now consisted of the wicker chair, the monkey ladder, and the flash cards and of course the balance beam and stepping stones, which she didn't really like and would sometimes protest loudly. Then slowly but surely with Bill and I holding her hands, she got used to it and didn't protest as much.

Pony Riding

ONE DAY during our well-earned coffee break, one of our young volunteers told us that a friend of his was doing a work experience course at riding school for young people with learning difficulties. His friend said that he loved the job and was hoping that the stables would make him permanent. When he told his friend that he was doing his Duke of Edinburgh award with us the friend suggested that maybe Catherine would like to come to the riding school? I asked him where the riding school was and he said it was in Lydiate.

Bill said that would be about a thirty-five mile round trip. I said that because our days were so full, I didn't think that we would have the time to fit it in but that, Bill and I would look at our schedule to see if we could manage it. Later that evening, Bill and I spoke about the riding school, and after working out how long each task would take us, decided that because the patterning table and the crawl box was out of the programme we could possibly fit in the riding school. Bill looked through his A to Z and found that we could take the Formby bypass, which would bring us to the area we wanted.

One afternoon Bill, Catherine and I set off to Lydiate to find the riding school. Eventually, after going round the roundabout a couple of times, looking for a sign to say there was a riding school nearby we found it at the bottom a leafy lane. We knew we were at the right place because we saw three little pony's and riders being walked around the field by some young people.

As we got out of the car, a woman in knee-high boots and hooded waterproof jacket came towards us an introduced herself. Her name was Mrs.Taurpy. There was a caravan on the side of the field and she invited us in and offered us a nice hot cup of tea, which was very welcome because there was a nippy early autumn breeze in the air. She said she hadn't been running the riding school very long and just recently she had applied for funding. If she was successful with the funding it would enable her to have a small indoor track for the riders and the volunteers so when it rains or it's very windy they can ride without getting wet or catching cold.

While drinking our tea a young woman came into the caravan and introduced herself as Mrs. Taurpy's daughter.

She told us she also worked at the riding school and supported her mother in all she was trying to do. After chatting and getting to know each other Mrs. Taupy said if Catherine would like to join the riding she would be very welcome. We were delighted.

So every Tuesday, weather permitting of course, Bill and I would take Catherine for her riding lesson, which she really enjoyed. She used to ride a beautiful little mild tempered pony called Christy. We still have a couple of photographs of her sitting proudly on Christy. In fact, she even got to the stage where she could pick her bottom up of the saddle and slow trot. There was always a volunteer at each side of her and one leading. Each rider had three helpers.

Sadly after a year or so we had stop going to the riding school because sometimes, if it was raining or very windy it could be uncomfortable standing around. Even though Bill and I could shelter in the caravan, Catherine would be outside and she was very prone to catching cold.

The Thursday Club

ONE EVENING a friend of Catherine's father came to see us. He told us that a club for young people with learning difficulties had opened in Garston. He said that his son Peter was a member and had made some new friends and his son absolutely loved going and maybe Catherine would like to join. He said the club met every Thursday evening from seven until nine. Bill and I thanked him for letting us know and said we would certainly take Catherine there the following week.

The next Thursday evening I got her ready to take her to the club. When we arrived, I was very impressed. One of the members came over to me and introduced herself as Kay. She told me all about the club. Then, after our introduction, I told her briefly about Catherine and how her accident and how sometimes she can get frustrated because she never regained her speech. She replied it was ok she understood. Then Kay asked would I like to leave Catherine to mix with the others and call back for her about nine? She told me not to worry because she would look after her. I readily agreed because I felt the genuine love and care from everyone who was there.

On our return, Kay said that Catherine had really enjoyed herself and she would look forward to seeing her again next week. Just before we left, I was introduced to one of the founders of the club. Her name was Lynne Lloyd and she had a daughter with learning difficulties. She, her husband Ken, and a group of friends from The Bridge Chapel in Heath Road, Garston, had decided to open the club for our special young people because there were no other venues available to them. Here in the Thursday club they could play music, dance, do puzzles, jigsaws, and make some friends.

It was up to the members what they would like to do because it was their club. I thought how fantastic! It was just what Catherine and many more young people like her need, to have a social club of their very own.

As time went by the Thursday club grew from strength to strength. So much so, that every year the founders and volunteers would take their members for a well earned break. Sometimes to Wales, and sometimes to Ribby Hall which is situated just outside Blackpool. They'd organised all the transport and accommodation and certain volunteers were assigned to look after some of the members like Catherine, who needed to have a one to one support. A doctor who was a member of the Bridge Chapel and Cathy, who was a qualified nurse, and a young mum with a young family, always accompanied them.

A week after their holiday we'd all be invited to go to along to the hall in Bridge Chapel and watch a film showing how everyone had enjoyed their holiday. It warmed my heart to see Catherine mixing with other young people who were just like her.

All of the volunteers, many of whom are teenagers, belonging to Bridge Chapel in Heath Road Garston, are wonderful and very caring people. They give their time selflessly to others and ask for nothing in return because they do it out of love. I never realised from that first introduction to Lynne Lloyd how much more secure Catherine's future would be.

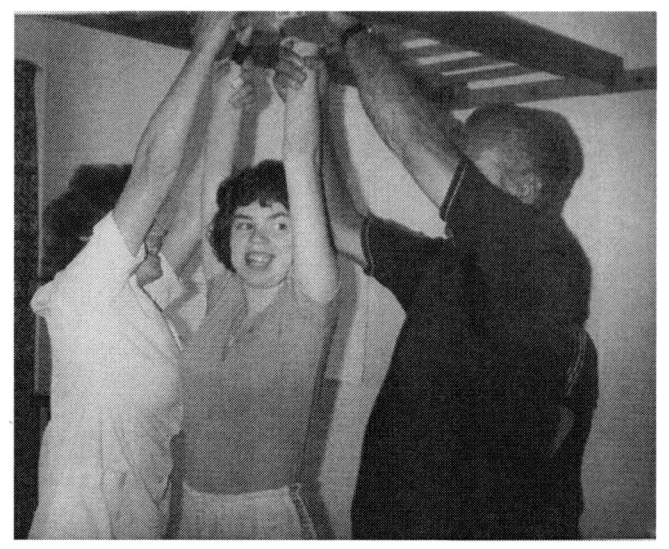

Therapy with Mum and Grandad

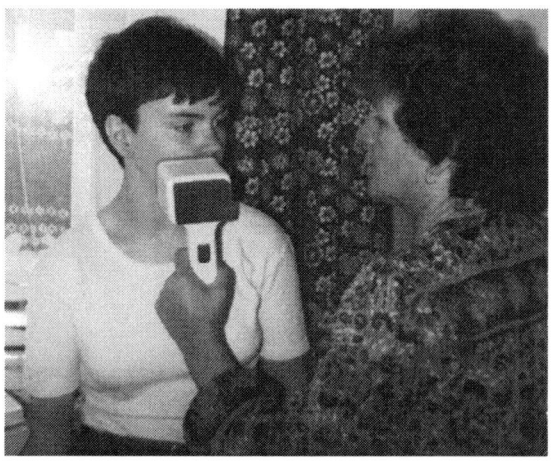

More therapy with Mum

28

Our Scary Journey

OVER THE third year on the programme, Catherine made another breakthrough; she had learned to drink from a straw, which was just fantastic! I was so delighted that every time she needed a drink I'd give her a soft drink and a straw; but sometimes I would be pushing my luck because she would protest until I gave her a cup of tea.

As we were returning home from her last assessment, we had a terrible experience. It was a beautiful sunny autumn afternoon as we drove away from the Institute in Somerset. I wound my window down and felt the cool breeze blowing gently on my face. I never liked the motorway because throughout the time we'd been travelling back and forth to Somerset for Catherine's assessments, we'd had couple of very nasty experiences because of some very reckless and carless drivers on the roads, so much so that I would find myself feeling very anxious when Catherine's assessment was due.

Even though the A roads took much longer, Bill always promised me before our journey that he would not drive on the motorway and he never did, bless him.

As we left the Institute, we drove directly onto the A38, which would take us through Bristol, Gloucester and Tewkesbury. Then we'd join the A449 in Worcester to take us through Kidderminster and Wolverhampton to pick up the A41 at Wolverhampton, which would take us to Whitchurch, on to Chester then onto the A56 where we would be just an hour away from home.

Bill and I had decided that once we got home we'd head straight to our local chip shop and get some fish and chips for our tea, because it would be late by the time we arrived home and I didn't fancy having to make a meal after our long journey so we were looking forward to that.

In the meantime, before we'd left Knowle, I'd been to the shop where my friend Dot worked and bought some snacks and canned drinks and put them on the back seat next to Catherine. Each time we travelled to Somerset for an assessment I'd ring Dot to let her know when we'd be coming. She and her husband George were always delighted to see us and looked forward to hearing of Catherine's progress.

As we drove out of Gloucester, the sun lay hidden behind the clouds. After about an hour on the road, we noticed that the sky had become grey and overcast.

We drove along a narrow country road where tall hedgerows cut out the light from the already darkened sky. Here and there were houses offering bed and breakfast, something that I hadn't noticed before in all the times we'd travelled those roads. Throughout our journey, the weather slowly began to deteriorate. By the time we got to Wolverhampton, dark patches of fog gathered here and there, which made visibility bad.

Suddenly and to our horror, we found ourselves enveloped in a fine blanket of mist. Bill drove very cautiously. I squinted as I tried to look though the murky mist, just in case I saw a B&B so that we could take shelter for the night. Visibility wasn't very good and everything and everywhere seemed so quiet. There was an awful eerie atmosphere.

I was beginning to feel anxious and felt we were lost. I didn't tell Bill how I felt, he was under enough stress and he didn't need me to lose my cool. As if he knew how I felt he said, "Don't worry babe we'll be home soon" His words didn't comfort me because I felt we were so alone.

As we drove, I kept talking to Catherine reassuring her that we'd be home very soon. Under my breath, I prayed. "Please God stay with us; help us to get home safely"

Then in the distance, two dim red lights appeared. They seemed to come from nowhere. Bill and I looked at each other. We were surprised but relieved in a way; at least it looked as if someone else was on the road, just like us. Bill said it looked like the back end of a truck, or maybe it was a local person who knew the area and was making their way home, so he decided to follow the lights. He said that the driver of the truck would be able to see a bit better because he would be higher in his cab and if that driver braked, we would brake. So we had no option but to take a chance and follow him. I don't know how long we trailed those dim red lights but I was too frightened to blink in case we lost sight of them.

After some time, which seemed like forever, we noticed in the distance that there were some murky lights ahead and as we drew nearer the lights grew brighter. A few minutes before, we had lost the dim red lights of the truck that we'd been following. Bill stopped the car and got out. We were amazed; those dim red lights had brought us onto the forecourt of a garage that was familiar. We'd arrived in Whitchurch on the outskirts of Chester. We both felt much better although we still had a long way to go. At least we now knew where we were. "Thank you God! Thank you." I repeated over and over.

I reached inside the car and brought out the canned drinks that I had bought in Dot's shop. Bill and I had a drink. I put a straw inside a can of lemonade and gave it to Catherine. Thank God, she had learned how to suck though a straw. After we'd rested for a few minutes and with a welcomed visit to the toilet for the three of us, Bill said it would be best if we got back in the car and made our way back home. We still had about thirty-five miles to go before we'd get home to Speke. The dim red lights that had bought us safely to the outskirts of Chester had gone.

Leaving the brightness and safety of the garage, we set off on the next hair-raising part of our journey. All the time Bill drove cautiously. After driving for a while we came to a roundabout; where thankfully, fog lamps enabled us to see a bit better through the fine mist and hopefully find the road we were looking for.

We strained our eyes looking for the signs of Helsby and Frodsham. After driving around a roundabout three or four times we saw the road sign that we wanted. No matter how familiar one is on certain roads they can look very different though the haze of the misty fog. Gradually we came to Helsby and the tall road lights threw a very welcome yellow glow upon the road. Bill and I just looked at one another and smiled "Getting nearer," he said tapping my knee. I looked over my shoulder to see how Catherine was. Her head was resting on the side window and she'd fallen asleep.

Then we saw the signs for Frodsham. Bill carried on driving. Through the thinning fog and in the distance we could see some lights. As we drove nearer, we could see the top of the Runcorn Bridge looming defiantly through the mist. Once safely over the bridge we drove though Halebank then on to Hale village. Then at last, we drove into Speke.

Bill drove right up the path straight to our front door. On hearing the car, our next-door neighbours came out to greet us. They'd heard on the weather forecast that a terrible fog had covered the part of the country where we were and we'd been in the thick of it. It had been foggy at home but not as bad. They were so pleased to see us and thanked God that we arrived back home safely.

With a deep sense of relief, I opened my front door and that took some time because my hands were a bit shaky. I stepped into the hall, turned on all the lights and looked about me. Bill was supporting Catherine because she was stiff and in pain from having to sit in the one position apart from her one trip to the toilet, since we'd left the Somerset eight hours ago. Both of us rubbed her legs to help get her circulation going. Then we wrapped our arms around each other, so relieved and thankful to having arrived home safely.

The chip shop forgotten, we settled for some tea and toast.

I felt that someone must have been watching over us. Those dim red lights sent to guide us to a place that we were familiar with, which would help us and encourage us to carry on with our journey. I also know my husband's skilful driving that brought us home safely. That was a journey Bill and I will never forget, so much so, that when I hear the weather forecast and there's a fog warning a shiver runs down my spine.

~ 29 ~

Four Years into Therapy

A WEEK after our nightmare journey we carried on with Catherine's programme. Each day was beginning to get a bit more difficult as she was protesting more and not really wanting to carry on; but after some coaxing and sweet talk she would co-operate so we would make the most of it. At least her programme wasn't as strenuous or as physical as it used to be and we didn't need the volunteers anymore; it was just Bill and I.

Of an evening after tea, Bill and I would sit at the table and try to encourage Catherine to write. The Institute gave me a special little holder that I could attach to the pencil so that she would have a better and stronger grip. Then I'd write her name and address, in dot-to-dot on a page of A4 paper and ask her to go over them and most of the time she did.

One evening, without writing the dot-to-dot first, I wrote her name and asked her to do the same. Then I gave her different piece of A4 and asked her to write her name, and to my amazement, she did. My heart was racing as I watched her. It was all wobbly but that didn't matter she did it! I took her face in my hands, kissed her, and told her how fantastic she was and she smiled and clapped her hands.

Every evening, and keeping our fingers crossed for the same results again, Bill and I went through the same routine with her with the paper and pencil. We began to take the dot to dot out of the writing, and sometimes it worked, sometimes it didn't. It was just separate words or maybe a small sentence. She couldn't write prose or compositions and I don't suppose that she ever would; but at least she was making an effort and she did it to the best of her ability.

When we went to Somerset four months later for our next assessment, we showed the staff Catherine's attempts at writing from the very first page. They were absolutely, delighted with her progress and so she had earned another achievement award for being able to control a pen and to write some single words. This was 13th November 1985.

The Programme Comes to an End

AS TIME went on Catherine became very difficult and she was beginning to refuse everything and anything to with her programme. During the time that she'd been on the programme, 1981–1986, she had made many significant strides. She was much brighter and more aware of her surroundings. She could taste her food and had stopped dribbling. She could pull out her tongue and she could suck though a straw. She could walk up and down the stairs without me with the support of a rail on one side of the wall. She was toilet trained, which meant she could go upstairs to the toilet and see to herself without me, but without her knowing, I would stand at the bottom of the stairs and listen, just in case of an accident.

She had begun to write her name and even though her writing was wobbly, she tried. When I read with her, she put her finger under each word and I'd ask her to say it, even though she couldn't speak she would make meaningful sounds, but sadly no speech. And of course the main thing was that the fits were getting less and less. After trying a couple of different medications, Tegretol was the one that seemed to curb her fits. The specialist at Walton Hospital was very pleased because it looked as if he found the medication that suited her. Bill and I were overjoyed because it was just awful watching her in spasm, writhing uncontrollably on the floor and feeling so helpless, but during her fit, she knew I was always there with her.

People who already have these skills may think that Catherine hadn't achieved or gained anything from her programme, but she had to start all over again and had made significant strides towards maybe and hopefully achieving much more. No matter how Bill and I tried to encourage her to carry on with her programme, she was adamant, she didn't want to do anymore and would sit and shake her head from side to side.

For a whole week, Bill and I tried to decide what we were going to do regarding the programme because it was getting very stressful for the three of us. By the end of that week, we made our decision. We had to respect Catherine's wishes. She'd had enough. She was twenty years old. I got in touch with the Institute and told them what had happened and what we had decided. They wrote back and said that they fully understood and would respect what we had decided to do and wished Catherine and us well for the future. And so another door had closed on another episode in my daughter's traumatic life.

During which time Bill and I were delighted to hear that that some of our volunteers, the ones who were aiming for the Duke of Edinburgh award, had achieved and received their well earned award and also a couple of our younger volunteers and gone to London to receive A Good Citizen award from champion swimmer Duncan Goodhuw. Well Done!

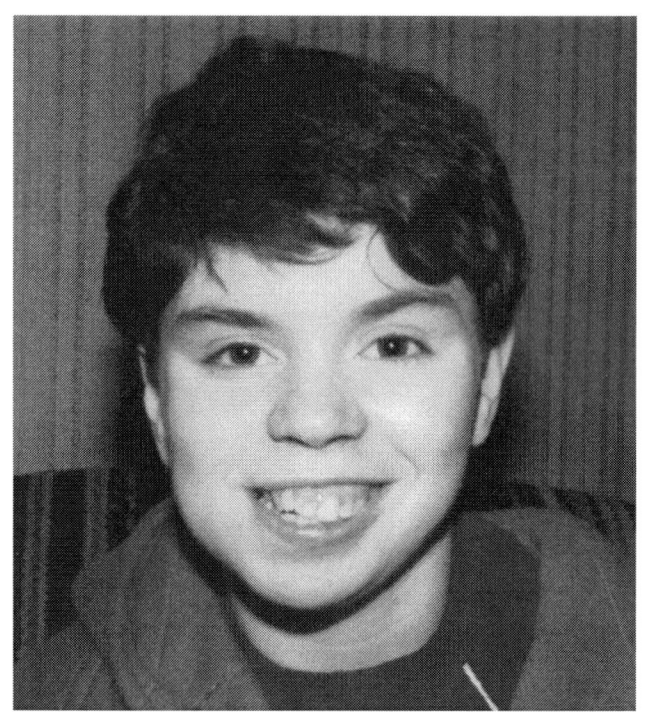
Catherine, age sixteen

~ 30 ~

The Day Centre

OUR LIVES had been so full over the last five years doing Catherine's programme we had to try to find out what we were going to do next. What was she going to do now? What was she going to do all day? She just couldn't sit in the house all day and do nothing. Then a friend of mine, who had a niece with learning difficulties, suggested that I get in touch with social services, which I did.

A couple of weeks after my phone call to social services, I received a call from a social worker; saying she'd like to come and see us regarding Catherine. When she arrived she had a briefcase tucked under her arm and an efficient look on her face, then she held out her badge of authority and told me her name. She was a social worker and had come to see how she could help Catherine.

I showed her into the living room and introduced her to Bill and Catherine. Once we had the introductions out of the way, we began to explain what we'd been doing over the last five years.

We showed her the photographs that Bill had taken of Catherine and the volunteers throughout the programme and the achievement awards that she had earned from the BIBIC. She was very impressed and she said that she had never heard of the programme before.

After hearing all about what Catherine's needs were, she said that the best thing to do was try to find her a place in a good day centre. We didn't know what a day centre was, but if it was anything like the little one that she used to go in Garston a few years ago that would be so great, but over a matter of time, and to our cost, we soon found out that it wasn't!

She said that day centres were especially for young people who had learning difficulties. She also said that the day centre wouldn't be able to do what we'd been doing, but could promise that she would be stimulated throughout the day by doing different sorts of activities and sometimes be taken on day's outings to places of interest. She also said that a special bus with an attendant on board would pick Catherine up at nine in the morning and return home at four. Bill and I were so pleased to hear that, it sounded just right. We knew Catherine didn't feel comfortable walking outside, she would go tense and begin to screech, but we had to try, and if it didn't work out we'd try something else.

Of course, we knew that the day centre wouldn't be able to do what we'd been doing, but at least she will be going out and meeting other young people who, like her, needed to be active and not left sitting in the house all day. Before the social worker left, she said that she would make an appointment for us to visit the day centre. She said it was only fifteen minutes by car from where we lived.

In due course, we received a phone call from the manager of the day centre who made an appointment for us. We looked forward to meeting her and seeing what they had to offer Catherine.

Our first impression of the day centre was that it was bright and clean. I noticed there were some photographs of some young people on the corridor wall whom I presumed where attending the day centre. I also notice that there were a few young people wandering about the corridor. I looked at Catherine and said, "What'd you think?" She just smiled back at me. We sat on the seats outside the manager's office and waited. About ten minutes later the door of the managers' office opened and the three of us went in.

The manager introduced herself to us. She said that the social worker had told her all about Catherine regarding what she could and couldn't do. She said that there was no way that they could give Catherine special attention. We said that we didn't expect that, we just wanted her to be doing something constructive while she was there. Time is very precious and like all of us she just couldn't afford to waste it.

It was arranged what day Catherine would be attending the day centre and where the bus would pick her up. Bill and I would take turns in taking her to the bus stop and collecting her from it. Some days she was fine but other days she would screech as we walked to and from the bus.

The ironic thing was that each day to get to the bus, we had to cross a Zebra Crossing, the same one that Catherine's father, myself and some of our friends and neighbours, who all had children at neighbouring schools, had campaigned for as Catherine lay in a coma just a few short years ago.

At first, everything seemed to be running smoothly and Catherine seemed her bright and cheerful self. Every morning one of us would take her to the bus stop and wait for the day centre bus to arrive. Then we'd do exactly the same when it was time to pick her up. The female attendant on the bus was usually bright and talkative and so was the driver. They grew to know and understand Catherine and she them, but if the attendant was off ill or on holiday and somebody else was in attendance, that would worry me a little because they wouldn't know anything about her.

As time went on, we noticed that when she came home at four o clock she seemed listless and not interested in anything, and after her tea, she would just sit and watch the television. Sometimes I would turn the television off and try to read to her but after a few minutes she would just push the book away. Then I'd get some paper and pens, draw some funny faces, and try to encourage her to do the same, but all she did was draw circles then push the pen and paper away. Her actions didn't seem right, well, I knew they weren't right. I needed to know what she was doing for the six hours a day while she was in the day centre.

I rang the day centre and asked to speak to the manager. I told her that Catherine seemed to have lost interest in some of things that she enjoyed doing. Like when I tried read to her, or tried to encourage her to do some writing or drawing with me and she hadn't wanted to know. All she wanted to do in the evening at home was just sit and watch the television.

Then I asked the manager how Catherine was getting on at the centre. After a lengthy conversation, she gave me what sounded like a favourable report. She said that it had taken some time for her to settle in, but over the last few weeks, she was beginning to join in with her group. She said that we must give her time and we weren't to worry. Then I thought, with naivety, that maybe, just maybe she had been busy in the day centre and was too tired to do anything else at home; how wrong I was.

~ 31 ~

Disillusioned

AS TIME went on we still didn't see any difference in Catherine, and she still didn't show any interest in anything. She seemed happy and content but I felt that she wasn't moving on and she didn't seem to be making any progress. It was just as if she was stuck in a rut, but not of her own making. I rang the day centre and asked to speak to the manager. The person who answered me said that the manager wasn't available now but could she help? I said that I would like speak to the person in charge regarding our concern over Catherine's progress, or rather the lack of it. I also said I had been in touch with social services, as I would like a social worker to see, as well as us, what Catherine does during the six hours a day when she's there. She said that was fine and made an appointment for us to come the following week.

When we arrived at the centre, we were taken into the managers' office. The man sitting behind the desk introduced himself as the new manager. Apparently the female manager who we'd met on the first day had resigned, which left him with staff problems. I think it was the escort on Catherine's bus who told me the present manager was leaving but nobody had mentioned when and we (parents) were not informed of this change.

I asked where Catherine was and he said that a member of staff had gone to fetch her. A couple of minutes later Catherine came into the office accompanied by a care worker. She smiled at Bill and me and sat in the chair between us. Just then, the social worker arrived all flustered and apologetic that she was late. Nevertheless, I was so glad she came because I needed someone from the council to hear what we were discussing and why. I told the manager what my first concern was. I wanted to know what Catherine was doing for the six hours each day that she was there.

In addition, was she getting the promised stimulation she needed? We would like to see a record of what she'd been doing for the past two years she'd been attending. The social worker interrupted and said that she also would like to see a record of Catherine's activities. We were delighted to hear that because I felt that at last someone was listening.

The excuses poured out. He said since the manager had gone many changes had taken place, and they were very short of qualified staff. He said that some young people were more capable of doing certain activities than others; so they had to be put into a different group so that they wouldn't be held back.

I said that I totally agreed with him about them not holding back other people; then I asked if Catherine was in that group? He said no, not at the moment, because they were still in the processing stage and they had quite a few young people with learning difficulties to process. The reason for this was because some young people with learning difficulties had just left their special schools and therefore needed a place at the day centre, and that is why they needed more staff. He also said that unfortunately he couldn't show us anything regarding Catherine activities at the moment; but her care worker would be back from holiday next week. I looked at the social worker and waited for her to respond.

She said that unfortunately, that was the situation for the moment, there were many young people with learning difficulties ready to leave their special schools and all of the day centres were in the same situation.

Then the manager asked would we like to make an appointment to come and meet Catherine's care worker when she returns from holiday. Bill and I just looked at each other. I think that we both felt the same way—let down. Bill stood up took Catherine by the hand and walked out of the office without saying a word. Before I left, I said to the manager that I would like to make an appointment to meet Catherine's care worker, as I needed to speak to her. He made one for me there and then. Before I left the office, the social worker wrote the time of the appointment in her dairy and said that she would also be at the meeting with Catherine's care worker.

As I walked over to the car, where Bill and Catherine were waiting a feeling of despair came over me. I felt so let down. All the hard work that Catherine and we had done seemed to be slipping away.

The following week we went back to the day centre to keep our appointment with Catherine's care worker. After the pleasantries and general introductions were made, I asked the obvious question. What did Catherine do while she was in her group for six hours a day? She said sometimes Catherine wouldn't take part in some of the activities that were offered to her. I asked if there were any alternatives for her when this happened.

She shuffled her feet, rubbed her hands together with embarrassment, and seemed to be lost for an answer. Then, as if a light had gone on in her brain, she said quickly, "Sometimes I given her some coloured pencils and paper and asked her to write something for me, anything." Then she said she would leave her and walk away to her other charges.

I asked her did she go back and look to see if Catherine had written anything. She said that after a little while she would go back and find that she hadn't done anything. I said it was no wonder that she didn't write anything because she, the care worker didn't show any interest. She was very indignant when I said that, she said that Catherine wasn't the only person that she had to look after. I replied that I was very aware of that, but Catherine's needs were just as important as the others were.

Then I said, "Don't you ever do any activities as a group so that everyone could join in? Like cutting up lots of card of different shapes and colour, and then make a game and see who can pick the right colour and match it with the shape. You could also do that with pictures of animals, birds, or fish, at least the group would be doing something that would stimulate them because they would have to think about which would be the right object. And another activity that you could try is the alphabet, which means making plenty of cards with letters from the alphabet a, b, c, etc, then the group could have fun picking out the ones which related to their own name, then try to put them together so it that it would spell their own name. Then when that person picks out the correct one everybody could clap and make a fuss of the person who got it right; which I'm sure would not only be stimulating but be good fun."

So after a promise that she would try to work something out, we left it at that and waited to see what was going to happen. The social worker didn't turn up at the meeting; but she did ring me that morning to say that she just wouldn't be able to get there as she had rather large work load. However, I was to let her know what the outcome had been.

A week or so later I received a phone call to say that Catherine had a new care worker, would we like to come and meet her. Bill and I hoped that this really must be a change for the better so we went to meet the new care worker with an open mind.

When we arrived at the day centre a member of staff took Bill and I to where Catherine was with her group. Of course, when Catherine saw Bill and I walk in the room she stood up and walked toward us. Then the young woman who was sitting in front of the group stood up and introduced herself as Cathy.

And I must say this was the cause of some laughter from the group. Cathy was the name of Catherine's new care worker.

She was a bright and bubbly young woman and we liked her straight away. After making sure that the rest of the group had an activity to do, she sat around the table with Bill, Catherine and I.

The first thing she said was that a cookery class was about to start the following week and she had put Catherine's name on the list. There were also some outdoor activities that she might like, such as going out on the mini bus and visiting different places of interest, which were for just one day a week, because this activity had to be shared with the other members of the day centre so that everyone would have the chance of a day out. Then she said that she had put Catherine's name down for the Friday afternoon club, which was at the British Legion in Netherly.

Then she asked would we be interested in the holiday scheme? I couldn't believe it, it sounded really good and positive. She said that certain members of staff would accompany the young people who were in their group while they were on holiday because they would know what their individual needs were.

I said yes course we were interested in the holiday, anything that kept Catherine on her toes and for her to be with some young people instead always being with Bill and I. It was just what we wanted for her. We thanked Cathy for giving us some hope and for sorting some kind of worthwhile stimulation for Catherine. Before we left, she said that the manager would like to have a word.

He asked us were we happy with what we'd been told? Bill said it sounded really positive and hoped that it would come to fruition, because we both knew that Catherine needed so much more than what she had been getting lately, and unfortunately time goes by so quickly, then he added, "We'll just have to wait and see"

He nodded his head and said that he understood our concerns and that from now on, every six months, we would have written report of how Catherine was getting on. Then he asked was there anything else he could do for us. I asked could the bus pick Catherine up from the house because sometimes she could be difficult and screech when she's out walking.

I told him that the screeching had nothing to do with the centre because she would be like that sometimes when we took her out. He said that he understood because sometimes Catherine could be like that when she's in the centre, so he made arrangements for her to be picked up from the house. Bill and I thanked him for his time and we left the centre feeling much better, but still with a little apprehension.

Thankfully, the bus began to pick Catherine up each morning from home and dropped her off, which was less stressful for the three of us. For the next twelve months, things seem to settle down. The following summer she went on holiday with Cathy and her group. She was also joining in some of the activities at the centre, not much but at least making an effort. I think that the highlight of Catherine's week at the centre was her Friday visits to the British Legion club in Netherley.

Over a certain length of time I found that the cookery class was beginning to sound like a joke because Catherine would bring the same note home each week which would read, "Could Catherine please bring in two slices of bread and a small amount of butter as she going to make toast"

Thoroughly fed up with same thing each week I sent a note back suggesting that they might try to be a bit more adventurous and try something else. Like adding a piece of cheese or maybe some baked beans, I didn't get a reply.

The problem was that she wasn't getting the attention that she should have been getting. When I'd mentioned this I was always told the same thing; there were so many young people with learning difficulties and not enough staff. I began to realise that no matter what we said or did we were fighting a losing battle.

32

Stepping Out into the World

TO SAY we were fed up with the whole thing would be an understatement. I decided to write to the social services at the main office in Liverpool. I told them about the day centre that Catherine was attending and I complained about the lack of stimulation and the sloppy attitude of some of the people who worked there. And as far as I could see Catherine was sitting there all day doing absolutely nothing! With the exception of going to the Friday club which was just once a week! She had lost some of the skills that we'd taught her, most of all her writing. Sometimes of an evening after tea, Bill and I would sit with her and try to encourage her to write but she would refuse because she'd got so used to doing nothing. A couple of weeks later we had a visitor from the social services in Liverpool. She said she'd come to see us about our complaint and to see what she could do to help.

Over a couple of hours, Bill and I told her about all the hard work that we'd done. All about the therapy, the volunteers, and how we'd raised money and how we'd travelled to Bridgwater every three months for assessments. Then, after doing all that, how we felt let down by the day centre, but worst of all, it looked like Catherine didn't seem to mind, or she may have thought, well if they don't care, I don't care!

We told her of the numerous meetings we'd had with the staff at the centre but to no avail. She understood our concerns and was very impressed with the work that we'd done. She said that she would arrange a meeting with a group of people whose main concern was finding jobs for people who had learning difficulties. These jobs could be from as little as two to three hours a week even a full week depending on their disability. Bill and I were delighted to hear this. It could be a chance to give Catherine the stimulation she needed.

In due course, we arranged a meeting with a group of people who were committed to helping young people with learning difficulties. Which meant they would help each individual person to find a meaningful job with a wage at the end of the month, which would also help them to mix more in the community? It was so refreshing from what we'd endured in the past.

Sitting around the table were six people, eight with Bill and I. As we chatted one of the group placed large sheets of white paper on one of the walls. Bill and I looked at each other wondering what they were for and were thrilled when we found out. As the meeting began we were asked what Catherine's' likes and dislikes were. How did she get on with people? How would she cope in certain situations? Did she dislike noise? Could she cope in a crowded room? As we answered the questions, one member of the group began writing our answers on the large sheets of white paper on the wall. They explained that they were building a profile of Catherine so that they could find out what would be best for her.

After some debating from the group, they decided a job in the Body Shop would be suitable for her. So they put one of the team members in charge of the task of applying for a job at the Body Shop in Liverpool city centre; explaining Catherine's disability of course.

I was totally unaware that these schemes of finding people with a learning disability work even existed. I wished I had known about it before, but there was no time for regret, the past was gone. At least something, more positive was going to happen now.

A few weeks later Catherine obtained a part time job at the Body Shop in Liverpool. She and her appointed support worker had their own little workroom where they filled the little baskets and boxes with beautiful fancy soaps, ribbons and other toiletries and she loved it. The other assistants in the shop were very nice to her and treated her same as their other work mates. Catherine's support worker picked her up from home by car and returned home teatime. It was only for two hours one morning a week but it was a start to better and bigger things. During the following year, the team found her another job because sadly her time at the job at the Body Shop had come to an end. The new job was in the admin dept at a local hospital. The hours were the same as the Body Shop but she would be able to stay there longer. I the meantime I had to keep her wage slips to show to the Social Security just in case it interfered with her benefit- which it didn't it was only two hours week. At last, it looked as if Catherine could look forward to some sort of future.

IN THE meantime, Bill and I began looking for an alternative to the day centre. Catherine was still going there but just for three days a week. Since I began badgering the social services I'd become quite an expert. Her social worker took us to visit two other day centres that we'd never heard of, but they didn't look any different to the one Catherine was already attending; too many people—not enough staff.

In fact, we did end up trying one of those day centres but Catherine was unhappy there. The staff said that when the group moved from one room to another—when they were going to do some craft work or some other activity Catherine would begin screeching and some of the group would get upset—so Bill and I decided that the best thing to do would was to take her out which we did. A friend of mine, who's neighbour had a son with learning difficulties, told me there was a small day centre opening in Croxteth, and maybe it would be worth my while to making inquires about it.

I rang Catherine's social worker, who seemed to put her all into her job and I thanked God for her she really did care about people; people like us who depended on her for her help and advice. She got Bill and me an appointment to go and have a look at the new day centre in Croxteth with a view to a placement for Catherine.

We had our meeting with the person in charge. She was a young woman with young staff who had some bright, new ideas for those who were going to attend. At the end of our meeting she said that she would like to come to our house and see Catherine in her home environment, which she did a couple of days later.

She sat beside Catherine on the couch and spoke to her. She asked her would she like to come to her day centre and make some new friends. Catherine answered with a big smile on her face. Before she left, she said that she would gladly accept Catherine. Bill and I were elated.

It was a small day centre and could only take 10–12 people. It was music to our ears. Catherine then cut her ties with her other day centre where she had lost some of her skills and which seemed to have done her more harm than good.

A few days later Catherine began to attend the new day centre. A special taxi picked her up at 8:30am along with some other young people who lived nearby; then brought her home at 4pm. She was much happier in her new environment and with her little part time job- and her future did look a little brighter.

In the mean time, I was finding it hard to cope with Catherine's daily personal care. As soon as I took her into the bathroom, she would screech and scream, which made the whole process of showering her very stressful. I got in touch with Catherine's social worker

She said that it was obvious that I needed some help and suggested I have allocated domiciliary care for one hour each morning. I was so glad to hear that, for as much as I loved Catherine, the trauma each morning was getting too hard to cope with. And so my domiciliary help arrived. Her name was Vera and she was a bright bubbly young woman and was just what Catherine and I needed.

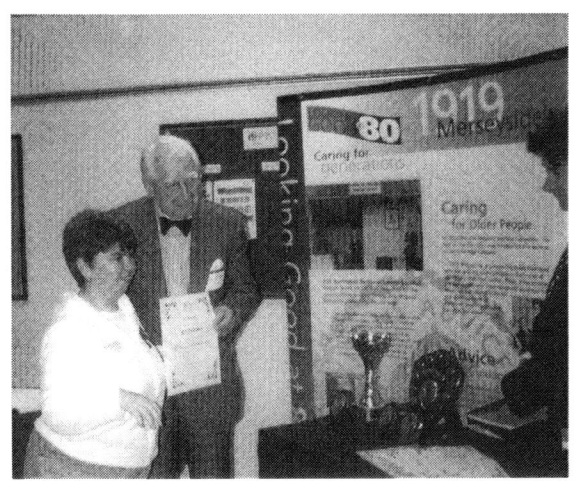

A proud moment for Catherine

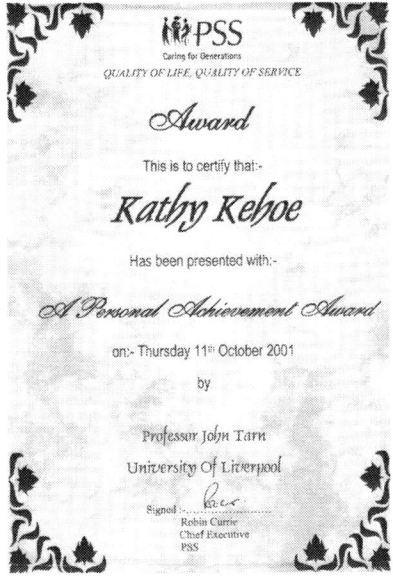

PSS
Caring for Generations
QUALITY OF LIFE, QUALITY OF SERVICE

Award

This is to certify that:-

Kathy Kehoe

Has been presented with:-

A Personal Achievement Award

on:- Thursday 11th October 2001

by

Professor John Tarn
University Of Liverpool

Signed :- ....
Robin Currie
Chief Executive
PSS

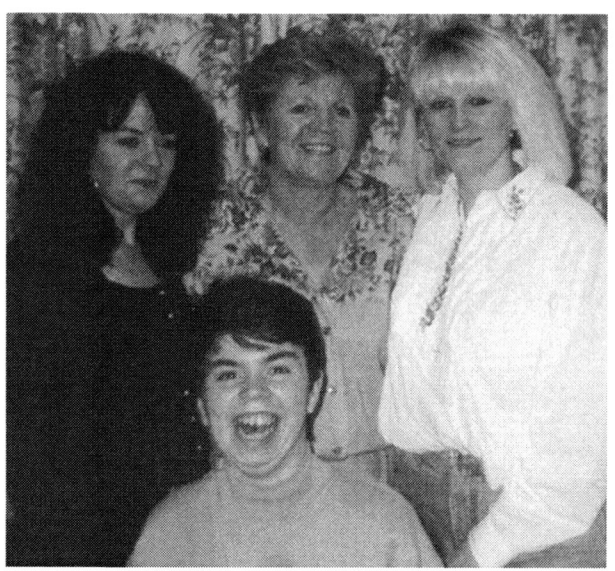

Catherine (center front) with her sisters, Julianne
(left), Christine (right), and her Mum

33

Letting Go

OVER THE years, Catherine's life has taken many twists and turns. After the therapy, she attended a couple of courses at Liverpool community college. One was a communication course with other young people with learning difficulties. We hoped it might help her communicate more because she couldn't speak but having said that, she communicates very well by pointing and making meaningful sounds.

Sadly, both of Catherine's part-time jobs and her community college placement ran their courses and ended.

Catherine enjoys playing ten-pin bowling, goes to the bowling alley every Friday afternoon with her support worker, and meets a group of friends there. However, best of all she loves going to the swimming baths with her armbands on, of course. She also loves music and going to the theatre, especially where there's singing and dancing on the stage.

Thankfully, she has experienced only one fit in the past fifteen years, after years of trying other medications, eventually; Tegretol worked. However, sadly, she never regained her speech; but having said that I still have hope that someday, no matter how badly, her speech will return. Over the years she has had some speech therapy but it wasn't very successful because sometimes she wouldn't co–operate with the speech therapist, or maybe it was because she just couldn't do what they asked. We used the Macaton signs, which were a much easier way of trying to communicate; she still uses some of the signs but not very much.

After a few years, some of the founders of the Thursday club had formed a group of trustees. Their aim was to buy a house or bungalow where three or four young people with learning difficulties could live independently but also with twenty-four hour support. Lyn Lloyd had told me some years before about what the founders of the club had had in mind and asked would I be interested. Because we'd been discussing our worries and anxieties of what would happen to our special sons and daughters when we're no longer around.

I said that I was interested as I was going to be seventy years old in the coming year (2008) and it would bring Bill and me some peace of mind to know that Catherine would be with the people she knew. And also the agency Natural Breaks, who were already supporting Catherine and Jenny, were still going to support them when they moved into their new accommodation.

In March 2008 Catherine and Jenny, who is Lynn Lloyd's daughter and another young woman, who all knew one another; went to live together in a beautiful sandstone bungalow in Allerton, which is only about fifteen minutes by car from where we live.

A few months later, when Catherine registered with a new doctor closer to her home, her support worker and I took her for her flu jab. I spoke to the doctor regarding the Catherine's epilepsy. I told him that thankfully she hadn't had a fit in nearly fourteen years and I was wondering if it would stay that way. I was concerned she may be taking unnecessary medication. The GP said that was wonderful to hear and felt that it wouldn't be very wise for him to take her off her medication, but, if he did it would take at least six to seven months because it had to be done very slowly. I said I would like to try it and if it didn't work of course she could go straight back on to it.

Then exactly six months, practically to the day when her medication was withdrawn, at 10:30pm on the evening of 15th August 2010 Bill and I were sent for. Because Catherine had had a bad fit and the staff had sent for an ambulance. I panicked and rang a taxi.

As Bill and I arrived at Catherine's bungalow, we saw the ambulance outside. The ambulance men were just wonderful and as she came around they took her temperature and blood pressure and thankfully, although she was groggy, she was fine. Her doctor came first thing the following morning and put her straight back onto her medication and ever since then thank God, she hasn't had a fit and takes her medication regularly.

Sadly as time went on the parents and the trustees decided that where the girls where living at that time wasn't really suitable and the other young woman had already moved out. So they decided to look for another bungalow. Eventually, after looking at a couple of other bungalows the trustees found just the one that the girls needed.

On 9th January 2012, Catherine and her friend Jenny moved into a charming dormer bungalow in a lovely part of Liverpool. It's a twenty-four hour supported bungalow, which is just what Catherine and Jenny need. Catherine needs assistance with her personal care like showering and dressing. She goes to the toilet herself and is independent in other areas.

She also needs someone to cook her meals and cut them up when needed because even though her taste buds returned and she can chew, she can't chew well. She sits at the table at meal times with Jenny and the support workers just like a little family.

Catherine is very happy and settled in her new environment and hopefully, the Lord willing, that will continue. Throughout the week she goes ten-pin bowling, swimming, house shopping and on a Tuesday she goes to a disco in Liverpool city centre which is only for young people with learning difficulties. The support workers are all bright, qualified and caring young women. Catherine and Jenny are well loved and cared for by the staff.

Bill and I will always be eternally grateful to the trustees of the Bridge Chapel, Heath Road, Garston, for providing a peaceful and secure home for Catherine.

One thing that I do know is that everything that the trustees do, they do it for the love of the Lord.

Every Wednesday and Saturday, Catherine and her support worker come to have lunch with Bill and me. Her family love her very much and if they can't come on the Wednesday or Saturday to see her because of work commitments they can always visit her at her own home.

Catherine's life is now full and as happy as it can possibly be for her. Because of this, I found over the last couple of years I have begun to feel a lot better and have accepted that when the inevitable happens, when Bill and I are no longer around, she will be safe in the environment that she is in now and she will always have her family to watch over her.

I must point out that I found it very hard to cope when the time came for Catherine to move out. The changes were so very difficult for Bill and I to get use to because we'd been so used to doing the same things together day after day; and it must have been the same for Catherine as well.

I found it so difficult having to go into her bedroom every morning to open the window as I always did and still do. Two chairs at the dining table instead of three, just Bill and I, but for the first couple of weeks I'd lay three places for dinner. Just shopping for two instead of three and if I saw her favourite thing that she loved to have, I would get very upset.

If Bill and I had an appointment at the hospital or dentist or such we would have to try and arranged the appointment to fit in between eleven-o-clock of a morning and no later than three o'clock in the afternoon. If that couldn't be arranged we would have to ask one or other of her sisters if they could be there when the taxi dropped Catherine off at home. We didn't have to do that anymore.

The worst time of course was when four o'clock came and Catherine didn't come home. Over the following months in fact, for a long time after she left, I felt as if I was living in a different world because three of us had always been together. Some days I would feel as if I was living in a different place.

I bought her a new bed and furnishing for her new home because I couldn't bear to part with any of her belongings. I felt so lost and so guilty; guilty because I just couldn't cope anymore.

She's forty six years old now. And it was forty years in June 2012 since the accident. She has slowed down a little but she still has her bright and happy personality. I ring and speak to her every morning and every evening. She speaks to me in her own way with meaningful sounds and with encouragement from her support worker. And she comes to see us twice a week because I just couldn't start the day without knowing she was alright.

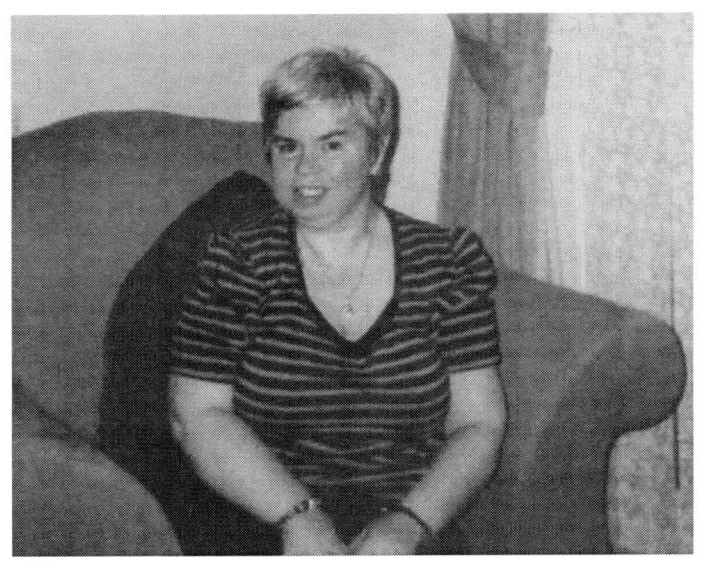

Catherine, Christmas 2012

34

We Count our Blessings

MY ELDEST daughter, Christine, works for Age Concern. Her job consists of looking after and caring for older people who have complex mental problems. On her days off, she is looks after her little granddaughter Jessica while her parents go to work. Jessica will start school this year. But now, I hope that this is the time for her to enjoy something that she has always been interested in which is counselling. My one and only beloved son Tony is an excellent joiner and can carve a piece of wood into a piece of art. He is also a very talented singer songwriter and writes all his own material. He holds workshops at Sudley House in Aigburth every forth Sunday where anyone and everyone who would like to recite a piece of their own written work, such as, songs, playing guitar and of course any budding poets. I must say the workshop is growing month by month.

Tony's wife Michelle, is a lovely and caring person and in-between working a fulltime job and looking after their two little daughters, she's kept very busy. Lily who is as beautiful as her name and who came late into our lives is a bright and intelligent little girl and is about to start her senior school in September 2012. Her little sister Ruby has a very creative mind so we have to make sure that we have a good supply of coloured paper, pens, stickers and paints. They both come for tea every Tuesday.

My daughter Julianne, is a support worker and works for the same agency who supports her sister Catherine. With her support work and in between helping look after her two grandchildren Lyla and Patrick, Julianne life's is very full.

Between Lily, Ruby, Jessica, and Lyla and Patrick, my little office looks like the Walker Art Gallery in Liverpool. But my paintings are far more artistic and far more valuable and made with so much love.

Our eldest grandson Antony, my daughter Christine's son, is an honest and intelligent young man and holds down a very responsible job. He is a logistics manager at a car plant. And his little daughter

Jessica is the love of his life.

Our granddaughter Julia is a beautiful articulate young woman who holds a responsible job in a bank as a data programmer. She is married to Simon who works for a Large Music Company and they have two children, a daughter Lyla and a son Patrick.

My youngest grandson Paul, Julia's brother, lives and works in Liverpool city centre; and is doing his best to live life to the full, as a young man should.

Bill and I are in our early seventies now and are in reasonably good health. Bill has angina and reoccurring vascular problems. Sometimes his arteries are blocked and he has difficulty when walking. He goes to the gym three times a week to do some special exercises because it's good for his circulation. His hobby is gardening, which he really enjoys. We have two large gardens, one in the front and one in the back, so in between doing odd jobs for the family he has plenty to keep him busy. In the back garden on one side of the fence, he's made five little birdhouses.

Every two or three weeks we go to Widnes market and buy bird seed, fat-balls and nuts to fill the feeders which hang in between the little bird houses. During the summer months, I bought a wrought iron birdbath and it's such a joy watching the birds taking a bath. We have plenty of blue tits, robins and a little bird that we believe could be a goldfinch; we also have thrushes and blackbirds that visit us. Then of course, we have the humble sparrow, and there are plenty of them. On the odd occasion, and not being far from the River Mersey, we sometimes get seagulls screeching and screaming as they fly overhead.

Bill feels so proud and delighted because now and again some of the birds rear their young in the little houses that he has made for them. He was especially overjoyed when some blue tits had begun to place some nesting material into one of the little houses and they reared their young there. Summer and winter no matter what the weather is like, he always makes sure that the birds have plenty to eat and drink.

I have arthritis, some days are good, and some days not so good, nevertheless I am in reasonably good health.

A couple of years ago my doctor gave me a referral letter for an induction at our local sports centre. They introduced me to Ricky who is a sports trainer at the Austin Rawlinson sports centre in Speke. Ricky was really, helpful and said there were quite a few people, men and women with arthritis and other ailments where exercise can help with mobility and give the participant sense of well being. Then he asked would I like to join his liveability class, which thankfully I did.

I've been going there for two years now and I must say its good fun because Ricky our trainer plays music while we do our exercises. It not only very good for your health it's where you can socialise and make few friends.

In the year of 2000 at the grand old age of sixty, I enrolled at Liverpool Community College. Over the two years that I was there, I took English, English literature, and Creative writing and I managed to get three GCSEs'!

My family were so proud you'd have thought that I had earned a first class degree, which proves it's never too late to learn. I was fifty before I learned how to swim, so that speaks for its self doesn't it?

When Catherine suffered that terrible accident, her father and I couldn't understand why. Why our little girl? We prayed so hard and so earnestly for her speech to be returned but it never happened. Nevertheless, her life was spared and we were so thankful for that. I vowed that no matter what her injuries were we would always look after her, which we did to the best of our ability. Nevertheless, it was too much for her father and as time went on he just couldn't cope anymore. On that terrible day when I found him dead in his bed I felt (but not at that time) that he'd been released from his torment. I will always hold a special corner in my heart just for him.

On the 11 October 2001, Professor Tarn from Liverpool University presented Catherine with an achievement award. She had been nominated for the award by PSS, Seel Street in Liverpool, who were the agency that supporting her at the time. Bill and I were so proud of her as she walked to the professor herself and accepted her award from him. Her father would have been proud of her too.

Now I look to what I have. My family have grown into responsible parents of whom I am so proud; five grandchildren and three great grand children of which I am equally proud. Proud of my children because as I gave myself and poured all of my energies into trying to get Catherine well again they might have felt neglected; so what I want say to them is, if they had ever felt that way and I'm sure they must have, I am so very sorry. But I was always there and had never left them. I love them with a passion as any mother loves her children; I still do and always will. Now that they are parents and grandparents themselves, I think that they may understand more of how strong and powerful the love you have for your child is and that's why I did what

I did for their sister.

All I can say is it could have been anyone of them on the terrible day in June 1972. I would have done the same for them because I love them all equally. The only alternative offered to me when Catherine had her accident was to put her in a home and let her wither and die, or take her home and do the best that we could for her and I chose the latter.

When I look back over the years and think of how Bill and I met, it was all because of my long time friend Sue. She was with me when I first met Tony when we used to go to the Dove and Olive when we were teenagers.

It was also because of her that Bill and I first met when she accepted two female tickets for the New Years Eve Party at the British Legion from Harry her neighbour. Sue has interwoven in and out of my life since we first met in 1953 when I first started work. Sue and Harry married in1979 but sadly, Harry died in 2007.

I've never regretted marrying Bill. Of course we have had our disagreements but we never allow them to last very long because whatever the disagreement was, it's always sorted out before the day is through. Each day and every day as we grow older together is very precious to us. I was right when I told my dad "I was as sure as the sun would rise tomorrow" about marrying Bill. Even today, we both still feel the same way about each other. In August 2012, we celebrated our thirty-second wedding anniversary.

When I look at Bill and remember how he came into our lives, I think maybe God had a hand in the plan and steered us together. I remember what my parish priest said to me many years ago. He said, "God show's his works through others." I didn't understand it at the time but I do now.

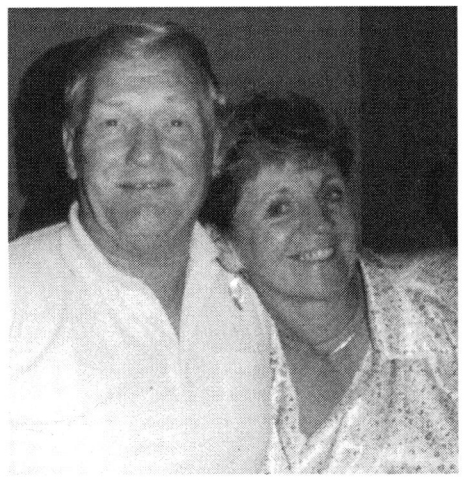

Julia and Bill